Towards youthful old
times together —
        much love,
        Gordon
April 17, 1975
Opening of
Old Timers'
Sexual Symphony

YOUTH
IN OLD AGE

YOUTH
IN OLD AGE

Alexander Leaf, M.D.

photographs by John Launois

McGRAW-HILL BOOK COMPANY
New York St. Louis San Francisco
Düsseldorf Mexico Toronto

Book design by Elaine Gongora.

Library of Congress Cataloging in Publication Data

Leaf, Alexander.
    Youth in old age.
    1. Longevity. 2. Hygiene. 3. Aging. I. Launois,
John. II. Title. [DNLM: 1. Aging–Popular works.
2. Hygiene–Popular works. 3. Longevity–Popular
works. WT120 L434y]
RA776.5.L38   612.6'8   74-20811
ISBN 0-07-036815-5

123456789KpKp798765

The author and publisher wish to thank Professor T.
Burrow of the Oriental Institute at Oxford University for
permission to quote from a conversation; W. H. Masters,
M.D., for permission to quote from Masters and Johnson:
Human Sexual Response (Little, Brown & Company, 1966);
and Sterling Publishing Company for permission to quote
from *The Guinness Book of World Records,* © 1974 by
Sterling Publishing Company, Inc., New York.

PREFACE

My first visit to the home of Khfaf Lasuria in the village of Kutol in the foothills of the Caucasus Mountains of Russian Georgia was in vain. After a long dusty ride over a very bumpy road we were greeted at her farmhouse by relatives who informed us that Grandma was off alone visiting friends at a distant village. However, my return a week later made up for this initial disappointment. Mrs. Lasuria was home and I had a long talk with this diminutive—she stands not five feet tall—sprightly woman who claimed to be 141 years old and who must be one of the oldest persons I've met, even though her stated age is surely exaggerated. She greeted our little party in warm Georgian fashion with toasts first with vodka and then with wine.

Although she carried a handsomely carved wooden walking stick, her nimbleness belied need of it. I think it provided a prop to enhance her distinctive dramatic poses for our cameras. Her memory seemed excellent as she recounted her first marriage at the age of sixteen; her husband died later during an epidemic of typhus and she married again when she was about fifty. A son, aged eighty-two years, lives in the stone house next to her. She described her concern when her first husband wanted to enlist in the army and fight in the Crimean War (1853–1856!). She told of her experiences as a midwife and of the hundred babies she had assisted into this world; of this fact she was very proud. She had time for several other careers as well, including that of housewife, collective farmer, and, quite recently, champion tea picker; she retired only two years ago. She sang with the Abkhasian choir of centenarians. The present was the happiest time of her life, she alleged, and with a smile and a twinkle in her eye she admitted unabashedly that she kept a bottle of vodka in her room and customarily started off the day with a nip before breakfast.

I came away from my visit with Khfaf Lasuria and her Georgian compatriots feeling that to live to be 100 was a most natural and simple thing. It took only a brief time back in Boston before that feeling was just another exotic memory. What fosters the existence of ten to thirty times as many centenarians per

100,000 of population in some parts of the world as in the United States? More striking and significant to me than the absolute ages of these elders was their remarkable physical and mental fitness and their obvious joy in life compared to the senility and debility so common among the elders of our society. What sustained these differences and what should be the role of medicine and the physician in researching the causes and aiding our elder citizens toward a more healthy, vigorous, and satisfying old age?

ACKNOWLEDGMENTS

Many have aided and abetted the production of this book, but only a few immediate contributors can be singled out for specific thanks. Dr. Miguel Salvador, cardiologist and leader of the team of Ecuadorian physicians who studied the inhabitants of Vilcabamba, graciously made available to me the results of his studies. Dr. Guillermo Vela, nutritionist, who was also from Quito, in Dr. Salvador's task force, provided his analyses of the local diets. Prefecto Clotario Espinosa of Loja Province, Ecuador, was a gracious host to us. Drs. Harold Elrick, Richard Erbe, J. Edwin Seegmiller, and authoress Grace Halsell were helpful coinvestigators on my second visit to Vilcabamba in 1974.

In Russia I owe special thanks to Professor G. Z. Pitzkhelauri, gerontologist of Tbilisi, Georgian SSR, for making available his own extensive epidemiologic studies of the elders of the Caucasus. Dr. Shota D. Gogokhia, the Minister of Health of Abkhasia, ASSR, assisted us in finding the old people scattered in their homes in villages and collective farms. I thank Dr. David S. Kakiashvili, Georgian cardiologist and gerontologist, for helpful discussions. Georgi Isalchenko, Director of Novesti, the independent news bureau in Moscow, and his colleague in Tbilisi, Merab Lordkhipanidze, provided important advice and guidance for our visit to the Caucaus. Igor Zakharov of Novesti served as guide and interpreter during our Russian visit.

In Hunza we were most grateful to the Mir, or King, Major General Mohammed Jamal Khan, for his warm hospitality and assistance with our work. Sultan-Ali, the headmaster of the single school in Hunza, was guide, interpreter, and friend during that visit.

Earle M. Elrick kindled my interest in longevity and supported my first visit to Vilcabamba. The editors of the *National Geographic* Magazine, particularly William E. Garrett and James Cerruti, arranged and supported our travels to the Caucasus and Hunza.

At home Dr. Norman Lichtenstein assisted with library research. Miss Sophie Katilus with limitless patience typed and retyped the many drafts of each chapter. My wife, Barbara, and daughters Caroline and Rebecca read and advised me on the text; I gratefully give them full credit for any portions which are good; for the rest I shoulder responsibility.

CONTENTS

maps of Abkhazia, Hunza, and Vilcabamba regions on page xx
photographs following pages 42, 98, and 164

INTRODUCTION

And lo! the starry folds reveal
  The blazoned truth we hold so dear:
To guard is better than to heal,—
  The shield is nobler than the spear!

Oliver Wendell Holmes (1809-1894), Songs in Many Keys,
"For the Meeting of the National Sanitary Association," 1860

It is significant that since antiquity medicine has been synonymous with the "healing arts." The art and practice, and—in recent times—the science of medicine have been highly personal. The physician has worked closely with the individual patient, who has sought him out to cure an already existing illness or pain. It is true that Roman emperors, as the Pharaohs of Egypt before them, did keep court physicians who were called upon occasionally to advise prospectively on matters which might affect the future health of the monarch, or to taste the royal food to ascertain whether it was poisoned. It was such a court physician who is alleged to have advised the Emperor Claudius that for health's sake he should dilute the wine half-and-half with water and that he should not suppress the passage of gas when the urge came to him, irrespective of the social setting at the moment. But such instances of preventive medicine were rare. Even with the scourge of the plagues and pestilences which wracked Europe during the Middle Ages and Renaissance it was likely to be the clergy or municipal authorities who instituted whatever crude quarantine or filth disposal measures were imposed. A responsibility of physicians for public health measures has been acquired only recently. It was the understanding of the relationship of bacteria and other microorganisms to human disease that came during the latter half of the nineteenth century which led to the control of infectious diseases through improved sanitation, immunizations, and, recently, the use of antibiotics.

Understanding the germ basis of infectious diseases in man led to the first widespread practice of preventive medicine. It had an enormous impact on our national health. In 1900 infectious diseases led the list and made up five of the ten leading causes of death in the United States, together accounting for 35.7 percent of all deaths. By 1968, of the infectious diseases only pneumonia and influenza remained among the ten leading causes of death and contributed only 3.6 percent of deaths from all causes. Life expectancy at birth at the turn of the century was forty-seven years and in 1969 the figure was seventy years. These figures constitute the measure of the enormous successes of preventive measures applied publicly to infectious diseases.

Further tightening of the control of infectious diseases is not going to improve our national mortality statistics appreciably. True, there remains much to be done in stamping out mortality from infectious diseases in underdeveloped parts of the world, but in the United States mortality rates from these conditions are already so low that further significant gains cannot be expected in this direction. Certainly venereal diseases are again rampant and need public measures for their control. Viral upper respiratory tract infections, the "common cold," claim annually a large morbidity, but the preventive measures for their control or eradication are either undiscovered or not feasible. Discomforting as they are, they do not cause deaths.

Reducing the mortality from infectious disease has simply uncovered another set of causes of death, as shown in Table 1. Heart diseases, cancer, and strokes now are the major killers. They affect mostly our elderly, and, as the percentage as well as absolute number of individuals over age sixty-five increase in our population, these conditions have preempted an increasing proportion of the physician's attention, time, and efforts. The engagement of the physician has been in the traditional one-to-one relationship with his patient, and the attention of the physician is generally sought only after a heart attack, stroke, or cancer has already made itself apparent. At this point the physician may help his patient to survive the acute threat, but usually he can do little to effect a "cure." The nature of these chronic degenerative diseases is such that they are often too extensive for the process to be reversed or cured by the time they make their presence known. A broader and earlier attack on these problems is needed.

With more than twenty million people in the United States over sixty-five today, the elderly comprise ten percent of the population—but they are the largest group in terms of medical need in this country. Although the resources expended on the health needs of our elderly form a large portion of the total national health budget (twenty-five percent of the ninety-four billion dollars spent in 1973 on medical care was spent on our citizens sixty-five years of age and older), the effects on increasing the life span have been miniscule. In spite of the increase in life expectancy at birth, from forty-eight to seventy years in the period 1900 to 1969, accomplished by reducing infant mortality,

TABLE 1
THE TEN LEADING CAUSES OF DEATH IN THE UNITED STATES IN 1900 AND 1969

Rank	Cause of death	Death rate per 100,000 population	Percent of total deaths
	1900		
1	Pneumonia and influenza	202	11.8
2	Tuberculosis	194	11.3
3	Diarrhea and enteritis	143	8.3
4	Diseases of the heart	137	8.0
5	Cerebral hemorrhage	107	6.2
6	Nephritis	89	5.2
7	Accidents	72	4.2
8	Cancer	64	3.7
9	Diphtheria	40	2.3
10	Meningitis	34	2.0
	1969		
1	Diseases of the heart	359.9	38.4
2	Cancer	160.0	16.8
3	Stroke (cerebrovascular disease)	102.6	10.8
4	Accidents	57.6	6.1
	Motor vehicle accidents	27.6	2.9
	All other accidents	30.0	3.2
5	Influenza and pneumonia	33.9	3.6
6	Certain diseases of early infancy	21.4	2.2
7	Diabetes mellitus	19.1	2.0
8	Arteriosclerosis	16.4	1.7
9	Cirrhosis of the liver	14.8	1.6
10	Emphysema	11.4	1.2

the facts reveal little change for the adult. Thus, an individual aged sixty-five in 1900 had a further life expectancy of eleven years, whereas in 1969 this expectancy was thirteen years—a gain of only two years. Medicine has thus far been unable to prevent or cure the chronic diseases which exact their toll on the elderly. Heart disease, cancer, and stroke remain the major causes of death of the elderly, in spite of huge increases in expenditures on the health care of the aged. Although acute coronary care units, organ transplants, coronary bypass surgery, artificial kidneys, etc., may provide brilliant solutions for a few fortunate individuals, they are incredibly expensive and generally unavailable to many who need them. There seems today to be no limit to the resources that could be consumed in trying to save the lives of individuals once stricken by these chronic ailments, with likelihood of only minimal success. Although the physician will continue to be charged by society with the obligation to care for the stricken, it is essential that a balanced attack be mounted— and that we appreciate that the only feasible solution to the problem is to increase our understanding of the primary causes of these chronic illnesses and prevent them from developing to the epidemic proportions which they now exhibit.

Because of the need to care for our stricken patients when the overwhelming concern is to save a life, medicine in the past decade has concentrated on the search for improved methods of sustaining life in patients with end-stage diseases. All of modern technology and medical science has been brought to bear on the problem. Artificial kidneys, cardiac pacemakers, membrane oxygenators (temporary artificial lungs), coronary bypass surgery, and even—briefly—heart transplants have resulted from this preoccupation. Cities have developed emergency teams to provide cardiopulmonary resuscitation, and hospitals have developed intensive care facilities for the care of such medical emergencies. In some such acute care units the costs of treatment may exceed $1000 per day. I don't decry the cost to save a life, but I simply want to indicate that at such a price facilities *cannot* be available to everyone who may need them. Furthermore, sudden death appears to occur in fifty to seventy percent of all deaths due to heart attacks. For some twenty percent of those dying suddenly, death is the first manifestation of coronary heart disease. A. B. Simon and A. A. Alonzo conducted a careful epidemiologic study of death in nonhospitalized cardiac patients. Based on the time of cardiac arrest and the call for emergency help, they concluded that no more than twenty-two percent of those in their study could have been aided even by mobile coronary care units. Thus the salvage rate is likely to be low, irrespective of the effectiveness of the supportive technology which may be available for the few patients lucky enough to gain access to an appropriately prepared facility.

Physicians have thus responded to the needs of their sick patients with an expensive technology and sophisticated specialization of knowledge that can save lives that previously were lost. Such a response is not inappropriate, but, in so doing physicians have focused increasing efforts, resources, and funds on the care of the individual. Effective as these measures may be for the individual, they constitute supportive rather than curative measures, and their availability will always be limited to the few "fortunates" who are stricken at the right time and place to gain access to the appropriate facility. The cost of such therapy increases exponentially as its effectiveness diminishes; that is, the sicker the patient, the greater the resources usually needed—but the slimmer the chances for success.

What is needed is a great effort to uncover the causes of these chronic afflictions and, simultaneously, to develop methods of prevention which will avoid the enormous difficulties entailed in their cures. Even when the physician and medical scientists discover the means of prevention, the implementation of the knowledge will undoubtedly require the participation of the general public. Unlike the situation with infectious diseases, in which a single agent is the cause of the illness and an immunization may be all that is required to prevent and control the disease, arteriosclerosis, the major killer today, is undoubtedly the result of a number of factors, the control of which will require continual vigilance. Even from the rudimentary understanding we now possess it is apparent that our whole life style may need changing, including diet, exercise, and work habits, if we are to attain a vigorous old age free from the infirmities and debility which plague many of our elderly citizens today. Medicine can search for the answers, but when they are found an enlightened public will need to adopt the necessary measures to assure continued good health and well-being.

In the fall of 1970, at the urging and with the support of a friend, Earle M. Elrick, I traveled with his brother, Dr. Harold Elrick, to Ecuador. There we visited the valley of Vilcabamba and examined the old people in that remote Andean village. What I saw of the old people intrigued me, as it seemed very relevant to health and longevity here at home. Later the editors of the *National Geographic* Magazine asked me to prepare an article for them on longevity. It was agreed that it should include observations and comparisons between three remote areas of the world reputed for the longevity of their inhabitants. In addition to Vilcabamba I visited the state of Hunza at the northern tip of West Pakistan and the Caucasus of southern Russia. John Launois, as expedition photographer, was my traveling companion, and together we visited Hunza in September and October 1971 and the Caucasus in June and July 1972. Our article appeared in the January 1973 issue of *National Geographic.* The response to this article has indicated a great public interest in the topic of healthy vigorous old age. This book is my response to that interest. Its purpose will be to summarize for the reader what is known of the aging process and of the factors which nurture the Khfaf Lasurias. It will be apparent that the topic of longevity can be approached positively today with the possibility for most of us to add vigorous, enjoyable years to our lives. No one, I believe, is interested in sustaining life in the limbo of senility and debility; but a vigorous old age free from illness with enjoyment of life is a worthy goal for medicine and merits the interest and attention of all. Many important questions remain to be answered and much research is needed, however, before we can provide a specific prescription to optimize health and longevity.

YOUTH IN OLD AGE

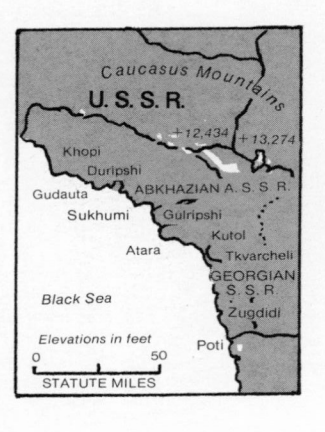

ABKHAZIA

Abkhazia is in southern Russis, in a region warm enough for farmers to grow tea and oranges.

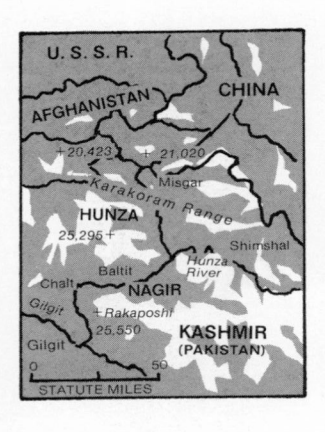

HUNZA

Hunza is one of the remotest realms on earth. Controlled by Pakistan, it is surrounded and protected by the huge mountains of the Karakoram Range.

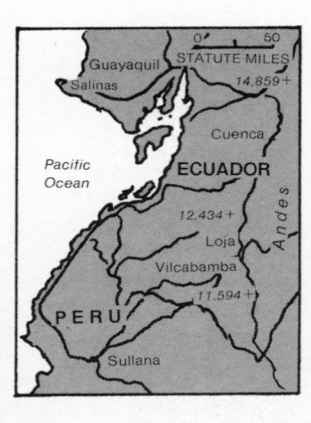

VILCABAMBA

For centuries, Vilcabamba has been isolated from most of the world. It is situated in the foothills of the Andes Mountains.

1

THE CAUCASUS

Grow old along with me!
The best is yet to be,
The last of life, for which the first was made.

Robert Browning (1812-1889), *Rabbi Ben Ezra*

Certainly no area in the world has the reputation for a long-lived people to match that of the Caucasus in southern Russia. As a student I had read of the famous bacteriologist, Élie Metchnikoff, and his hypothesis that it was the fermentative agent of yogurt, which was responsible for the unusual long lives along the shores of the Black Sea. It was, therefore, with great eagerness that I met my traveling companion and expedition photographer, John Launois, in the London airport where we boarded our flight to the Soviet Union.

In contrast to the remoteness and isolation of the two other places we visited, Hunza and Vilcabamba, the Caucasus has been on the main road to history. This mountainous area in southern Russia stretches across the land bridge from the shores of the Black Sea on the west to those of the Caspian Sea on the east. This land bridge has constituted a route by which civilizations have moved from west to east and vice versa. The Caucasus region today consists of the three Soviet socialist republics of Georgia, Azerbaijan, and Armenia.

Whatever isolation the Caucasus can claim today is bureaucratic rather than geographic. For months before my trip I had corresponded with physicians and gerontologists in Russia, but when the time arrived to obtain my visa from the Soviet consulate I was still unsure of the exact places I would have to visit in order to see the old people. I had hoped to call first on gerontologists in Kiev and Tbilisi to learn from them exactly where we should visit. To obtain a visa, however, one must present coupons purchased from the Intourist Bureau for hotel accommodations for each day spent within the Soviet Union. There is no such thing as an "open" coupon. Thus, after much thought, I made the best guesses I could as to where we wanted to be and when. Reservations were made and coupons purchased from Intourist on this basis.

The day after our arrival in Moscow, as we talked with officials of Novosti, the independent Soviet news bureau, it became clear that my "guesstimates" were not realistic. I found the Intourist Bureau anything but receptive to my request for a change in

3

travel plans. The gist of several days of confrontation was essentially as follows. They asked, "But if this isn't where you wanted to go why did you make the reservations and pay for the trip?"

I explained, meekly at first but with increasing exasperation, "There was no way that I could know where I needed to go until I arrived here and could obtain advice from gerontologists and others as to where the old people were."

Reply: "Surely you must be very stupid indeed to have purchased a trip you didn't want!"

In all fairness I could perceive a kernel of truth in that statement until I pictured the cold, official response in the Russian consulate in London: "I am sorry, but regulations are 'No prepaid reservations and tickets—no visa."

Finally, after paying a fine of several hundred dollars for changing our itinerary, we deleted Sochi from our schedule and added the time to our visit in Sukhumi on the Black Sea in Abkhasia. This proved to be only the beginning of the changes we needed in travel plans, each of which was fought to the finish (of our dollars) by Intourist. As a result of this obstruction it turned out that, in the five weeks we were in Russia, there were only thirteen days that we were working in the field. Most of the other time was spent in frustrating wrangling with Intourist over our travel arrangements. Even appreciating the fact that hotel and restaurant reservations for tourists are limited in parts of Russia (in order to plan appropriately they need foreknowledge of how many visitors their facilities will have to accommodate), they seemed an unusually hostile organization. Furthermore, their facilities seemed to have a degree of flexibility depending on one's willingness to pay extra.

In Moscow we picked up our interpreter and assistant, Igor Zhakarov, from Novosti, and—after an evening of excellent ballet—we started early the next morning for the airport. The flight to Tbilisi was bumpy, as we skirted a thunderstorm most of the way. The plane was full and flew within the clouds rather than above them, and seat space was cramped. The plane, a twin-motor jet, was quite old, but we arrived in Tbilisi safely.

Tbilisi is the capital of the Georgian S.S.R. In the daytime the city looks run-down, with dirty, peeling walls of buildings and untidy gardens. It does, however, have trees lining the streets, palms and birches, and at night by street light it is quite lovely. Igor and I went for a walk after supper at the Hotel Everia (the ancient Greek name for Georgia was Iberia). Almost the first building we came to was the opera house. In two minutes the curtain was going up on the evening's performance. We got two tickets at 1.50 rubles ($1.80) each and sat in a box for a most enjoyable performance. The opera, *Dusk* by Zachariy P Paliashvili, is a true Georgian production which premiered in 1923 and probably has been performed nowhere else.

The next day we pursued some sterile leads with one of the physicians with whom I had corresponded prior to our visit but whose cooperation terminated with our arrival. The following day we made contact with Professor G. E. Pitzkhelauri, director of the Institute for Physiology and Pathology of Women and a leading Georgian gerontologist. He proved to be most informative and generously shared his findings and views with us.

There are 4500 to 5000 centenarians in the Caucasus according to the 1970 census, we learned. In 1939 only 0.8 percent of the population in this region was older than sixty years. According to the latest (1970) census the figure had increased to twelve percent, with 1844 over 100 years of age in Georgia alone or thirty-nine centenarians per 100,000 of population. These are mostly concentrated in several parts of Georgia. In Georgian Abkhasia, which has 294 centenarians, the ratio was sixty per 100,000, but in the district of South Ocetenskaya the ratio was 103. The Republic of Azerbaijan has a higher average ratio than does Georgia, with eighty-four per 100,000.

Two-thirds of the old people live in small villages and the majority of these are at an altitude of 1500 to 4500 feet above sea level. Thus, they do not live at high altitudes but in a very hilly terrain. Western Georgia with its humid, subtropical climate has many more centenarians than does the eastern part of the republic, which is also hilly but drier. Centers of industry have the lowest percentage of centenarians. Professor Pitzkhelauri told us this was due to pollution of the environment. But industry has come only recently and factory jobs are more likely to attract the young from the farms rather than the very elderly. We also were told that the water was important for longevity; but chemical analyses of water in relation to the distribution of the elderly have not yet been performed by the Soviet gerontologists, who have kept busy documenting the ages of the elderly and their living habits.

Of the 12,000 Georgians over the age of ninety, one-third are male and two-thirds are female. The same ratio applied to the

1844 Georgians over the age of 100: 614 males and 1230 females. It is generally true that, among the very elderly, women out-number men some two to one. In the United States the ratio of female to male centenarians is two to one. Interestingly, there are slightly more boys than girls born in the United States, but the ratio reverses at age eighteen and from that age on women outnumber men with the inequality increasing with age. In the United States recent figures show that of the 6200 Social Security recipients claiming to be 100 or over, 71.5 percent are female and 28.5 percent male. Thus, upward falsification of ages of males in Georgia could not be a prevalent practice unless women were doing the same. Professor Pitzkhelauri believes women live longer because men use more tobacco and wine and are subject to more trauma and accidents. Other Georgians explained that women were biologically stronger than men. But when asked the evidence for this claim, we were told, "Because they live longer than men!"

Documenting ages is not always simple in the Caucasus. In the central portion of Georgia the religious background is Christian and church records are therefore available in some instances, but in Abkhasia on the shore of the Black Sea the religion has been largely Moslem and written records are rarely available. Professor Pitzkhelauri explained the methods he used to validate ages:

First, documents of dates of birth are given highest credence. Church birth and baptismal records are the main documents, but others are also useful. These include passports, papers such as letters, and sometimes writings or even carvings on doors and walls that record a birth in the family.

Second, age at marriage (usually well remembered), time until the birth of children, and the present ages of these offspring, which can usually be more easily verified) offer evidence of age.

Third, recollections of outstanding events such as war service, changes in the Tsarist regime, the Russian Revolution, the Russo-Turkish War, or outstanding local events—such as a drought or the unusually heavy snowfall in Abkhasia in 1910—are useful chronological markers.

We asked how reliable are the results obtained from the latter two approaches. Professor Pitzkhelauri replied that 704 centenarians whose ages were known from birth records were also tested by the questions. The results showed that, for nearly ninety-five percent of those tested, the questionnaire gave the same age as that indicated by the birth record. For most of the remainder, the correct age was within five percent and not more than ten years off the mark in any case. It seems probable that for those whose correct ages were known and validated by independent objective evidence a more accurate age would be obtained by the interview technique than would be expected to result from the latter technique alone in the absence of birth records. Even with an appreciation of the tricks our memories can play on us—deceiving us into believing that we have actually experienced events which we only heard of at an impressionable, early age but often spoken of by parents or elders—one can with an intelligent subject produce fairly convincing proof of age.

In the village of Kutol in Abkhasian Georgia we visited Khfaf Lasuria. This sprightly lady promptly gave her age as 141 years—the oldest we encountered. (The oldest living person was alleged to be Shirali Mislimov of Azerbaijan, who claims to have been born in 1805 but whom we were not able to see. He died September 1973 at the stated age of 168 in the village of Barzavu in Azerbaijan, west of the Caspian Sea.) According to Lasuria's account, her father lived to be 100 and her mother 101 or 102. She was the youngest of eight sisters and three brothers and the only survivor at the time of our visit. She had always lived in this village. She married her first husband when she was sixteen years old, but he and her one son by this marriage died in separate epidemics of typhus. She married again when she was fifty years old and had a second son after a couple of years, she told us. She appreciates the fact that her son was born to her late in life. (We heard, however, of other instances of childbearing by women in their late forties or early fifties, and evidence was presented later at the Gerontology Congress in Kiev of a delay in the age of menopause among the long-lived women.) This son, Tartuk, is now eighty-two years old.

Thus at the time of our visit in 1972 we arrive at an estimated age for Mrs. Lasuria of 134(50 + 2 + 82). At the time of the Turkish Wars (1873–1878) she was already married to her second husband, she claims (50 + 94 = 144 years old). Her second husband died twenty-eight to thirty years ago, and he was over 100. She was two years older than he (100 + 29 + 2 = 131 years old). When she was about twenty years old her village heard of a "big war in the north." Her first husband thought of leaving to serve in the army at that time. The only war "in the north" in those times would have been the Crimean War of 1853–1856 (118 + 20 = 138 years old). The very heavy snowfall of 1910 she remembers as a recent event. "My son was already an adult, then about thirty, and I was about seventy at that time." She remembers a snowfall of over two meters and of helping her son remove snow from their roof (70 + 62 = 132 years of age)—although Tartuk, aged eighty-two, comes out ninety-two by this estimate. She said she was seventy-five to eighty years old at the time of the Russian Revolution of 1917 (77 + 55 = 132 years old). She has been smoking since her favorite younger brother died in 1910. "He was more than ten years younger than me, and he died when he was about sixty" (60 + 10 + 62 = 132 years). In a *Life Magazine* article of September 16, 1966, Peter Young describes her, "Lasuria Khfaf," as being 125 years old then, though no basis for this age is stated. She is readily identified by a photograph in that article. Mrs. Lasuria doesn't remember her birth date, but she knows she was born in the spring of the year. She was told her age by her parents when she was fifteen years old and says she has kept count of her age since then.

Since the estimates are largely of minimal ages, it is difficult to argue with Mrs. Lasuria's claim that, "After the spring of this year I am in my one-hundred-forty-first year." Our interview was conducted in a manner that would have made it very difficult for each of these assessments to come out in such fair agreement unless a common thread of reality linked them. One doesn't achieve certainty by such a technique, but after repeatedly encountering similar consistent responses from other centenarians I have arrived at a degree of confidence that prompts me to place Mrs. Lasuria's age close to 130. In the absence of written records this is my best estimate, and it should be regarded as only that—an unverifiable estimate.

When we first called on this delightful old lady she was off visiting relatives in a distant village. Later she described a pleasant visit. She simply gets on a bus alone and goes visiting. She retired from the collective farm two years ago and has received a pension only during this time. In the 1930s and 1940s she held the record as the fastest tea leaf picker in her collective farm—and she was over 100 then! She considered herself young until five years ago. She smokes one package of cigarettes daily and inhales, a habit she has had for sixty-two years. She drinks a glass of wine before her noon meal and each morning before breakfast has a glass of vodka. She spoke lucidly and easily about events recent and past. At the age of seventy-five to eighty as a midwife she assisted more than 100 babies into the world. "I am very proud of that." She described the life of women: "Women had a very difficult time before the Revolution; we were practically slaves." And she ended our talk with a toast, "I want to drink to women all over the world . . . for them not to work too hard and to be happy with their families."

We had been forewarned that in Russia the ages of males were frequently falsified. This practice was based on an effort to avoid draft into the Tsar's army in the past, as the period of conscription was twenty years! However, according to the 1970 census, of the 1844 individuals over 100 within Georgia, 614 were males and 1230 females. Once again we find the 2 to 1 ratio favoring women.

As I have been frequently reminded, application of actuarial tables would indicate an exceedingly low probability of any human being living to 130 years. The longest documented human life, according to the 1973 edition of *Guinness Book of World Records,* is 113 years, 124 days, by Pierre Joubert, a French-Canadian bootmaker, who was born on July 15, 1701. It is estimated that the probability of attaining a lifespan of 115 years is only one person in 2.1 billion. The probability of exceeding this figure is of course, even more slight. Such calculations are based on life tables compiled in our advanced industrialized countries where extensive records have been kept, and of course the yardstick appropriate for one population should not be applied to another. The assumption that such a transfer can be made excludes the very possibility of a community wherein people live to ages beyond those which occur in the "advanced" industrialized countries. Thus, such calculations can give only the probability of attaining unusual longevity in the advanced industrialized countries which provide the tables.

Although such calculations cannot be used to exclude the possibility of unusual longevity cropping up in other cultures, neither do they help us to establish such occurrences. *The Guinness Book of World Records* introduces its section on longevity with the following warning: "No single subject is more obscured by vanity, deceit, falsehood and deliberate fraud than the extremes of human longevity. Extreme claims are generally made on behalf of the very aged rather than by them.

"Many hundreds of claims throughout history have been made for persons living well into their second century and some, insulting to the intelligence, for people living even into their third. The facts are that centenarians surviving beyond their

110th year are of the extremest rarity and the present absolute
limit of proven human longevity does not admit of anyone living
to celebrate a 114th birthday. . . ."

One would deservedly be characterized as gullible not to heed
such a warning. On the other hand there is no reason to be
certain that the absolute limit of human life has been demonstrated. What is needed, all will agree, is documentation, and
nothing is likely to substitute for the credibility which written
records can provide; but it would be a narrow view to conclude
that in cultures where such records have not been kept there may
not exist the conditions for longevity. Most of the populations of
the earth have, at least until recently, lived in societies with
deficient birth records or none at all. *The Guinness Book of
World Records* recounts, "The most reliably pedigreed large
group of people in the world, the British peerage, has, after ten
centuries, produced only one peer who reached even his 100th
birthday. However, this is possibly not unconnected with the
extreme draughtiness of many of their residences." Another view
might be that their record is excellent considering that they were
peers. Advantages of somewhat better sanitation, perhaps less
exposure to epidemics, and better nutrition may have abbetted
this group, but wealth, opulence, opportunity for self-
indulgence—as well as the "extreme draughtiness"—may have
had the opposite effect.

Unfortunately, there is no known method of distinguishing
chronologic age from physiologic age. That some persons age
much earlier than others is common knowledge. Presented with
two individuals exhibiting equivalent evidence of aging there is
no parameter—no blood test, no changes in bones or tissues—
measurable in these two persons which would allow the scientist
to distinguish which of them is the older chronologically. It is even
doubtful that such objective criteria may be forthcoming. Certain large molecules in our bodies undergo spontaneous cross-
linking as a function of time. Thus, the degree to which such
molecules are linked together might provide an internal clock by
which ages could be established. Collagen, the major protein
molecule in connective tissue, comprising some thirty percent of
all tissues in our bodies, is one such molecule that undergoes
cross-linking with time. It has been suggested that the solubility
(or other property which depends on the degree of cross-linking)
of collagen obtained from a small biopsy of skin might serve as
such an internal clock, since the degree of cross-linking increases

by one percent per year. Whether the degree of cross-linking is affected by other factors in the micro-environment which may differ in the individual who ages prematurely as compared with a "normal" individual is not known. Radioactive elements decay with a constancy which is, under usual conditions, independent of environmental factors, but chemical reactions, such as cross-linking of collagen, are generally very much influenced by the immediate environment in which they occur. Thus, it is likely to be a vain hope at present that any body constituent will provide an absolute measure of the passage of time.

We will remain dependent on records to document ages. Clearly, therefore, no absolute reliance can be placed on ages which have been estimated by such indirect methods as those we applied in the case of Khfaf Lasuria. But I am unwilling to discount ages such as she claims on any a priori arguments. Since I first reported my visit to the Caucasus in the January 1973 issue of the *National Geographic* Magazine, there has been considerable criticism of the advanced ages cited and comments on my gullibility by distinguished gerontologists and biostatisticians. Some of this criticism I must now admit to be justified. Old people do often exaggerate their ages. In 1970, when I first visited Vilcabamba, the oldest person in that tiny Andean village was Miguel Carpio, who then claimed 121 years. On revisiting Vilcabamba in 1974 I was startled to find the villagers claiming an age of 132 years for Carpio—a generous increase for the intervening four years! The last visit I had more time to study the baptismal records of Vilcabamba from which I can now conclude that Carpio cannot be older than 110 years—still a venerable age but not in excess of documented limits for the human life span.

It is noteworthy that the interest of gerontologists in absolute ages is rather different from mine. Since most, if not all, persons die of some specific disease, it is not known whether there is some biologic limit to our life span. This is a matter of great interest to gerontologists. My interest is, rather, to find societies where a large proportion of elder citizens retain their faculties, are vigorous, and still enjoy life. This difference in our interests in longevity, of course, does not give me license to accept and report exaggerated ages. Certainly I don't believe the 168 years that the Soviet Press claimed for Shirali Mislimov or other such extravagant, undocumented claims. However, one hundred years ago probably less than one-tenth of one percent of the world's population was keeping written records of births, so it may be a long, long time before the needed documentation is available; by then ways of life will have changed greatly every-where, perhaps in directions not so conducive to longevity. Therefore, I will present the ages of the individuals with as much accuracy as possible, based on the documentation or interrogation that was available. Fortunately we are not as concerned here with determining the limits of human longevity as with determining whether health, vigor, and enjoyment may accompany old age, rather than the debility and senility seen so commonly in our society even at much younger ages.

The figures Professor Pitzkhelauri provided for the activity of the elderly of Georgia are encouraging in this regard. Of 15,000 elderly over the age of eighty, more than sixty percent were still gainfully working, mostly on collective farms. Sixty-four percent were totally independent in their personal care, twenty-nine percent partly dependent, and seven percent needed assistance. Forty-five percent of these elderly go for long strolls daily out of their gardens, twenty-four percent walk from one village to another, twenty-five percent walk only in their house or garden, and the remaining seven percent are inactive, remaining in bed. Thus over seventy percent continue to be very active.

Fifty-two percent of those over eighty years of age were judged in good health. Only seven percent were ill. The remaining forty-nine percent had minor degrees of weakness or memory loss which were not incapacitating. The nature of illnesses was listed as follows: cardiovascular disorders were most important and affected forty-one percent of those who were not well; respiratory disorders, such as bronchitis and emphysema, affected sixteen percent; disorders of the nervous system and sensory perception affected eleven percent; urological disorders, 7.6 percent; intestinal disturbances, 5.6 percent; dermatologic and muscle disorders two percent. There was alleged to be no cancer and no syphilis, but a few chest x-rays showed minor evidence of tuberculosis.

When I asked doctors in Georgia of what did the old people die, I received a number of improbable answers. Some had theories that beyond a given age people are no longer subject to cancer. As far as is known there can be no basis in fact for such an assertion. There is, in contrast, every indication that the incidence of cancer in our society increases with age. The same would be the expectation in the Caucasus, but the fact is that there are no reliable data on the causes of death. The old people live and die in their scattered mountain villages and since they die in their homes there are very few autopsies. Without autopsies the cause of death is largely guesswork. Clinically we can usually accurately make a diagnosis of sudden death from heart attack; but without autopsies the real cause of death may be overlooked, particularly with cancer of internal organs, which may masquerade under a variety of clinical guises. Thus, the claims that cancer does not afflict the very elderly must remain questionable pending autopsies. The fact that they have attained old age, however, must mean that they have avoided cancer at earlier ages or that the rate of the spread of cancer in these old individuals must be very slow. Then, too, there may be an immunologic basis for such a situation. An immunologic reactivity which may be favorable to a long life, according to one theory of longevity, may also simultaneously provide an inhospitable setting for a cancer.

The response to my repeated question, "Of what do the old people succumb?" that most amused me was "Well, they just get bored with their long existence and decide to die!"

After much talking about the elderly, it was with great anticipation that we drove from Tbilisi to Mykheta, the ancient capital of Georgia, where we met Gyorgi Nikolai Garseveneshvili, who was born in 1880. He states that he now has a good life with a monthly pension of eighty rubles (about $100). Even if he "were twenty, life would be better now." He was married once, when he was thirty and his wife now is eighty. He had one daughter aged forty-five years. As a soldier before the revolution he fought under Nicholas II in the Ukraine against the Austrians. After World War I there was a bourgeois government in Georgia, and he fought against the Turks until 1922. He became an independent farmer after the fighting was over and later joined a collective farm, caring for the animals—sheep, pigs, and cows. He retired at age eighty-two and has worked about his home since then. He drank heavily—up to six pints of wine daily—but stopped five years ago. He doesn't drink vodka or smoke.

Garseveneshvili attributes his long life to nourishing food, hard work, fresh air, and a quiet and enjoyable life. He has good friends. He added: "Look after the girls when you can; but now I can't." His eyesight and hearing are good, and he doesn't use glasses even now. He recalls a fever once long ago, but, when I asked if he sees a doctor, he replied, "Why should I?"

He thinks the younger generation is much freer and better

educated than his generation. As a youngster he believed in God; now he no longer does, but he still goes to church for the major festivals. When asked what was the happiest period of his life, he replied, "I feel joy all my life but was happiest when my daughter was born and saddest when my son died at the age of one year from dysentery. I will enjoy the remaining years if God gives us peace." His blood pressure was normal at 118/60 and his pulse was regular at 70 per minute. A normal resting pulse is 60 to 75 beats per minute but somewhat slower in conditioned athletes. A normal blood pressure is 110 to 140 systolic and 60 to 85 diastolic.

In the village of Ichalto, near the town of Telavi and half a day's drive from Tbilisi, we met Nikolai Gyorgi Papalashvili, who was 103 years old and a farm worker born there. He can't remember the year of his marriage, but he married late. Church certificates validate his age. He was the youngest in his family; two sisters and three brothers all died at ages sixty to eighty-five. His parents lived to be over ninety and his grandmother lived to be 120, we were told. He has one daughter, age sixty, and one son, age sixty-three, both of whom are teachers in Telavi.

He remembers an impoverished childhood. When he married and built his own home, life began for him. He started school at eighteen and attended for five years in a neighboring village. He is proud, however, that just seven years ago he graduated from a local people's university—this was a two-year course of study with classes meeting twice monthly for the first year and once monthly the next year. Ichalto boasts the oldest academy in Georgia, and it is claimed that Shota Rustaveli, the national poet, was educated here in the twelfth century.

Papalashvili married his wife when she was very young and has lived with her for seventy years. He attributes his long life to the proper balance between work and rest, the good air and climate also being important. He drinks moderately but stopped smoking at age sixty, "because if I smoke, I'll die soon." He smoked only ten to fifteen cigarettes a day, although when he was drinking he smoked much more. The only time he was ever ill was when soldiers were being recruited to fight in Turkey. But he does worry now about his eyesight. He always has been strong and robust and always has enjoyed himself—but most of all from ages thirty-five to fifty, when he danced well and was "the best guest." Singing and dancing were his main hobbies, and he can still dance after a few drinks.

Roman Ytmeledzhe of Telavi, age ninety, is a stone en-

14

graver—the third generation of stone engravers in his family. His father and grandfather both died at eighty-five, and his Greek mother at eighty-three years of age. His first wife is living at age seventy-two, and they have four children, one son and three daughters, with ten grandchildren. He states, "Working hard and eating little are the secrets to a long life." He drank heavily as a youngster and now when he has company he drinks a lot (as we witnessed), but otherwise, when alone, he doesn't drink. He never smoked. The best period of his life was from thirty to forty years—"lots of women then," he added with a smile. His hobby is hunting birds and hare, which he still does in season. We were proudly shown his double-barreled shotgun, stamped "London," and at least as old as he.

We watched Ytmeledzhe engrave Georgian letters on a marble tombstone, which he did masterfully with a hammer and chisel, free hand. He works rapidly without glasses and is paid thirty kopeks (36 cents) per letter. He took us to the local cemetery where he proudly pointed to examples of his handicraft. Most of the past village notables and his friends now rest under his headstones.

With typical Georgian hospitality Ytmeledzhe insisted that we come to his home to share food and drink. All the family joined with the daughters and younger women at the table, but his wife and older female relatives did the serving. This was one of our first exposures to the incredible hospitality of these warm and generous people. Quickly the table was piled high with fresh greens, tomatoes, cucumbers, wonderful crusty homemade white bread served while still warm, roasted chicken, tangy sheep cheese, chicken livers and shashlik, spices, and finally fresh fruits—cherries, strawberries, and peaches, which were in season. This was washed down with a vast quantity of home-brewed wine, drunk with much toasting. The old man outdid us and in the end had too much—as did we! The young women contributed to the festivities by playing the piano or violin, or singing and dancing with skill, pleasure, and a total lack of self-consciousness. We departed with small gifts of pottery, feeling very jolly and warm indeed.

In the nearby village of Gurdzhany we met Mikhail Mchedleshvili, age 95, who still works on the collective farm from 5 A.M. to noon. He was a prisoner of war in Berlin until the Armistice at the end of the First World War. He was married before the war to his only wife and had one son and two daughters. He said he didn't know to what he could ascribe his long life, but working in the fresh air, being physically active, and having enough rest he thinks important. He drinks three to four glasses of wine with meals; he has never smoked. Both his parents lived to be over 100 and kept their teeth. One brother died at eighty and one sister at eighty-six.

Mikhail Mchedleshvili has always been thin. During the First World War he had very little but can't say that he had not enough food. Now he goes to bed at nine or ten and is up at sunrise. He was happiest when his daughters were born. Singing has been his hobby, but he hasn't sung for the two years since his son died. The greatest event for him was the Armistice and his return home. That gave him "a new birth." On examining him I found his resting pulse to be 120 with frequent irregularities and his blood pressure very high (260/124). There was a loud heart murmur transmitted to the neck vessels, which were quite dilated. He gets short of breath now with exertion but had no swelling of his ankles and no shortness of breath waking him at night.

In the course of examining the old people I found a broad spectrum of cardiovascular disorders. Unfortunately, it is impossible on a single visit to learn whether Mikhail had had high blood pressure for years or whether this had developed recently and I was observing the terminal stage of his disorder. His wife Anna, age ninety-two, also had high blood pressure but had a regular pulse and no other symptoms.

Mikhail's neighbor, Gyorgi Gvelykashvili, age eighty-seven, joined us and the two disappeared into the cellar of Mikhail's house. We followed and saw that the earthen floor was pock-marked with small patches of fresh earth partly covered by a flat rock. We watched with interest as the two old men selected one site, removed the flat stone, dug away the fresh earth with their hands, revealing the rim of a large wine vat. We were told that the large earthen vats, in this case eight, each had a forty gallon capacity, and were buried beneath the cellar floor so that only the rim would project above the level of the floor. Mikhail carefully scraped off the dirt that covered the lid, brushed off the lid, and carefully lifted it so that only a small quantity of soil fell into the wine. He then took a gourd dipper fastened to a long pole and dipped out several glasses of wine, which of course we had to try. The wine is fermented each fall from the juice of crushed grapes, and it is this juice which is then placed in the earthen vats to ripen. Each house seemed to have its own wine cellar and its own private vineyard. Satisfied as to the quality of the wine, Mikhail filled several pitchers before replacing the lid and carefully covering it with earth and its marker stone.

In the nearby village of Virgini we visited Sachro Mosulishvili, age ninety-three, and his seventy-four-year-old wife. He was born here and always worked in the fields and vineyards. He was head of the municipal council and founded the local collective farm in 1927. He served twenty years on the municipal council and twenty-four years on the collective farm, retiring in 1966. He was a soldier from 1901 to 1904 and was drafted again in World War I. For fifty years he smoked two to three packages of cigarettes per day but has stopped; he drinks regularly but moderately. He has had high blood pressure and in 1964 had a stroke, which left him with weakness on his right side. Since then he has reduced his drinking. His father lived to eighty and his mother to ninety. He had six brothers and two sisters. He has two sons by his second wife; his first wife was sterile, so he divorced her and remarried in 1922.

Mosulishvili enjoyed his youth more than any other time of his life as he was healthy and strong. He would like now to be young again, as his youth before the Revolution was very difficult. When asked to what age he regarded youth to extend, he stated, "up to fifty." He told us a man "must remember one good thing and one bad thing in life." For him a good year was 1921 when Georgia became free and liberated. The bad memory was that of life before the Revolution when he was virtually a slave. He attributes a long life to normal work, no smoking, no suffering, adequate rest, and a moderate amount of wine. He then added, "and one should eat a lot of green vegetables." He insisted that we try some of his wine and in short order a table was set in the cellar; beside the wine vat were shelves lined with preserves and white earthen jugs. His wine seemed especially good, but unfortunately our doctor-guide stood up and proposed one last toast to our host, put his earthen mug down firmly, and said, "We must go."

We then went to visit a ninety-five-year-old man and his wife, age eighty. There were many relatives present, and the meeting started rather coolly until an accordian was produced and the music livened up the gathering. The man, Karum Utiashvili, and his wife Keke, were soon joined by a neighbor, Kita Kandiashvili, age 105, and his wife Elo, age ninety-nine. There was a brief controversy between the two couples as Kita argued that he should have played host, as he was the older of the two. Nevertheless, we were taken up to the veranda where a table was quickly spread, and we sat down to the usual groaning board with the long flat bread, cucumbers, tomatoes, onions, garlic, slightly sour sheep's cheese, roasted and boiled chicken and mutton, salt, green peppers, spices, sauce, and wine. The initial toasts were drunk with homemade vodka or a Georgian brandy, the first a real firewater and the latter the pride of the Georgians. After these amenities, the drink changed to local wine and the toasting settled down to a steady pace throughout the meal—which, if allowed to run its course undisturbed, might continue from three to five hours.

Every person and every honorable and friendly sentiment provided an occasion for a toast. We were at first surprised that the Georgians invariably drank to Stalin; but he remains a national hero to them, even when the mention of his name in the rest of Russia is taboo. The drinking-glass tumblers were promptly refilled as the old people, ourselves, our driver, our parents, our children, peace, friendship, and understanding were separately toasted. Anyone who passed the house while such a feast was in progress was promptly seated at the table, and, while his character and qualities were extolled, he became the focus of renewed libations. Our doctor-guide was elected president of the table by acclaim—"empty your glass if you approve his election," we were told. Then he served as toastmaster, deciding the order of toasts and who might propose them. We watched with awe as, after proposing a series of toasts, the toastmaster might accumulate five tumblers of wine, which he would then drink down ostentatiously in rapid succession and continue with the merrymaking. This went on and on and on before we finally broke away. The next morning proved that the natives were much hardier than we were!

We saw several other individuals in their late nineties before we returned to Tbilisi, but we were eager to see the centenarians, and Abkhasia seemed to be the place to do so. Our battles with Intourist, however, were not over. We wanted to go directly to Sukhumi to see the centenarians. However, our itinerary had been changed once in Moscow, and Intourist didn't want to change our travel plans again. After much wrangling, arrangements were made for us to travel to Sukhumi three days later. The time meanwhile hung very heavily on our hands until we could leave Tbilisi. We were feeling intensely frustrated and restless in not being able to visit the centenarians and get on with our work. However, we found a chessboard and passed many pleasant hours with its help.

The flight from Tbilisi to Sukhumi was only some fifty-five minutes, but time enough after our forced idleness to considerably raise our spirits. The temperature was seventy, with balmy breezes, and the town with its many vacationers had a festive air. We took a boat ride and swam in the Black Sea, which further refreshed us. After a lean seafood supper we turned in early with hopes of getting quick cooperation from the necessary officials in order to start work in the morning.

The next morning we had a visit with the local minister of public health of Abkhasia, Shota Gogokhia, who proved to be highly cooperative and helpful during our stay in Abkhasia. It was, however, the weekend, and therefore impossible to arrange any interviews, so we visited a new resort town, Pitzunda, north of Sukhumi. On our return we found an invitation to visit Dr. Alexander L. Grigola, who was born in 1879. He was professor of health resources for Abkhasia and had retired one year ago. His daughter, also a physician, says that in the past year he had suffered from the idleness of his retirement. Having chopped all the necessary wood for the winter and dug up and replanted the whole garden, he had nothing further to do. He told us that he had graduated in medicine from the University of Tomsk with high honors; he became interested in public health and returned to Abkhasia to make a study of health conditions and the environment. After the Revolution the local governor asked him to continue his work and make Abkhasia world famous as a health center. At that time there was much indigenous malaria, tuberculosis, and dysentery in the region. Dr. Grigola opened the first sanatoria in Abkhasia by converting a prince's estate and then a monastery to that purpose. He states that there were centenarians before the Revolution, but there were few individuals age sixty to ninety. (The 1939 census figures had indicated that only 0.8 percent of the population was older than sixty years of age.) Since measures were taken to eradicate malaria in the 1930s and other public health measures reduced dysentery, tuberculosis, meningitis, venereal disease, etc., the proportion of individuals older than sixty years greatly increased (to twelve percent in 1970) and now more centenarians exist.

Dr. Grigola's father died at age ninety; his mother died of

meningitis at forty. One sister died at ninety-three and one aunt at 105. When asked his recipe for a long life, he replied, "The first and last thing is to preserve your nervous system and control your emotions." When asked how one does this, he said, "I don't know. I never managed to learn that myself."

The next morning we were driven to the collective farm at Duripshi where we were introduced to a delightful trio: Markhti Tarkhil, age 104; Temur Tarba, age 100; and Tikhed Gunba, age a mere ninety-eight. All were born locally.

Temur had just had his one-hundredth birthday on May 20, three weeks before our visit, and it was apparent from his bearing and happy manner that he had "arrived." His father died at 110, his mother at 104, and an older brother had died just that year at 109. Temur smokes a good deal but doesn't inhale. He continues to work on the collective farm, cultivating maize and tea. He was decorated a Hero of Labor by his government only seven years ago. This highest civilian decoration was awarded in recognition of his work on the cultivation and hybridization of corn. He still devotes the mornings to collecting tea and working in his garden. One of his seven children and his first wife died, but his second wife is now seventy. Temur's blood pressure was a youthful 120/84, and his pulse was regular at a rate of 69. While I was checking pulses and blood pressures the other two would shake their heads in mock sadness at the one being examined and remark, "*Plokho, ochen Plokho!*" ("Bad, very bad!"). This friendly clowning went on all day. Temur seemed in excellent spirits with a sharp clear mind and a good sense of humor.

Markhti Tarkhil also proved to be a sturdy fellow. However, because of redness and dryness of his conjunctivae, he appeared older. His parents died when he was young and he was raised by a grandmother. Both grandparents lived to be over 100 years old. He had worked as a farmer all his life and has bilateral Dupuytren's contractures (a permanent limitation in extending the fingers) from his rough physical work. He told us that when he was born his grandmother poured cold water over him and now he swims daily in a cold mountain stream regardless of the season or the weather. We were witness to this. Climbing into the car we drove toward his swimming place, until the road became impassable. As we stood about arguing with the driver whether the car could or could not make it over the ruts, Markhti started off independently, staff in hand, to walk down the steep rutted dirt road to the river below. It proved a difficult half mile, but Markhti moved quickly and agilely over rocks and down the river bank. I hurried after him, trying to keep alongside in case he should tumble or slip. Familiar with the thin and fragile bones of our elders, I was terrified that he would fall and, at the rate he was moving, surely disintegrate. The skeleton, just as do the muscles, loses minerals and mass with disuse, and hip fractures, often heralding the beginning of the end for the unfortunate oldster, all too frequently result. Later I learned from the regional doctor that there is no osteoporosis among the active elders, and fractures are very uncommon.

Having arrived at the river bank, Markhti stripped and waded into the stream where he lay on his back splashing the cold water over himself. Our young guide from Moscow then stripped and waded into the stream too as it was beastly hot and the brisk walk had us all sweating. But the water was too cold for Igor, and he promptly returned to the bank. Being an old polar bear type myself I also tried the water. It was fine but very cold—I would estimate some 45° to 50° F. After bathing, Markhti scrambled up the bank and dressed again in his several layers of clothing, topped off with his full woolen tunic, riding pants, and high boots, and climbed back up the hill to the car.

Markhti's wife died years ago, and he thinks of remarrying "for fun." He has never been fat and eats everything with no special diet—meat (except pork), butter, cheese, vegetables, fruits, and grains—but he eats less now. Aside from having had malaria when a young man, he has never been ill and has never been in a hospital. He still goes annually to the high Alpine pastures. We found that during the summer months goatherds take their flocks to the tops of the low Caucasus Mountains to pasture, as they do in the Alps. During this time they live in the open with their goats in a very rustic but wholesome existence. Farmers have been exempt from serving in the army, so Markhti was never a conscript; but he fought with the militia when the Turks invaded Abkhasia. He remembers Tsars Alexander III and Nicholas II and saw the latter in nearby Gagra when the Tsar visited relatives there.

As was not uncommon in Abkhasia, Markhti did not eat pork. This is a residuum of the Moslem tradition. In the past Abkhasia was under Moslem domination. Now there is little religion and the three old men are all agnostics. Later we overheard a conversation in which Markhti said, "Although I don't believe in God, still I don't want to be buried like a dog with no ceremony when I die." There followed a discussion about the possibility of reactivating the Church, but Temur said, "Who needs it but you old people? No one will go but you."

Markhti attributes his long life to "God," to the mountains, to a good diet—and he warns against eating without pepper! His "best" age was eighteen, but he agreed with Temur that he regarded himself as a young man until the age of sixty. "I still feel young, I sleep well, ride my horse, eat well and swim every day, so I still feel like a youngster, though not so strong as I once was." When asked whether he still likes girls, Markhti rose and said, "Come, I'll show you!"

The third and youngest member of the day's trio was Tikhed Gunba, age ninety-eight. He was married when he was thirty and had eight children—one son was killed in World War II and one daughter died. His father died at age 125, he told us, and was one of the oldest persons in the region. (Markhti remembered him well.) Life was at its best for him when his children got married and when World War II ended. Tikhed doesn't smoke, but he drinks lots of wine. He eats everything but pork. He still works on the collective farm, picking tea and gardening around his own home.

Tikhed's blood pressure was 104/72 and his pulse was regular at 84. He seemed a very placid individual with much "mileage" left. In the presence of the two centenarians, it was evident that Tikhed was still regarded as a youngster.

We were invited to lunch at Tikhed's home. It proved to be a true Georgian feast lasting from 2 to 5 P.M. and enlivened by unmatched hospitality and warmth.

I had been told that the citizens of Georgia were the richest in material goods in the Soviet Union. Driving along the poorly paved roads, often swerving or stopping to avoid chickens, swine, or cows, I had the impression of traveling through an underdeveloped country. However, within their homes the Georgians live very well. Ostensibly good communists, they remain ruggedly independent. Toasts regularly included one to Stalin as their native son and hero, although his name is no longer mentioned elsewhere in Russia. Our young guide and interpreter from Moscow was continuously arguing with the Georgians; the bickering was evidence of the antipathy that exists between the Georgians and other Russians. Many of the elderly Georgians told us how much better off they had been since the Bolshevik Revolution. Their lot has improved greatly upon liberation from the feudal system and upon the enactment of subsequent agrarian reforms. But, in spite of the loyalty which the new regime in Moscow evokes and their splendid defense of the homeland against the last German invasion, Georgians are not above exploiting their particular social advantages. Agriculture remains their major means of livelihood and they are joined together in large collective farms; but these are not state farms. The work is performed collectively, but their produce is sold to the Soviet government on the open market and the income is divided among them—this is in contrast to the state farms on which the workers are paid a salary by the state and the produce is the property of the state. In a situation in which the agricultural programs of the Soviet government have lagged behind national needs, the Georgians have done very well in the prices they have exacted from the government for their vegetables, grains, fruits, and meats. When the government price does not suit them, they bring their produce to the local open markets and dispose of it privately. Such private markets flourish, and one can find almost any agricultural product in season for sale. The prices, however, seemed very high to me. Fresh tomatoes in season were selling for one dollar a pound. The Soviet Government has been largely helpless to control this expression of private enterprise; and many Russians feel the Georgians are robbing the state, while many Georgians disdain the tight-fistedness of their northern compatriots. Georgians are the colorful Texans of the Soviet Union.

By the time the "luncheon" broke up, the sun was already setting and it was too late for further investigations. Our spirits, however, were lifted by these playful old youngsters, and we were happy to be back at our interviews after the tedious delays of the preceding eight days.

2

HUNZA

In ancient times the people lived (through the years) to
be over a hundred years, and yet they remained active
and did not become decrepit in their activities.

Huang Ti (The Yellow Emperor) (2697–2597 B.C.), *Nei Ching Su
Wen*, Book I, Section 1 (translated by Ilza Veith in *The Yellow
Emperor's Classic of Internal Medicine*)

had never heard of the state of Hunza until a few years ago when one of my patients, concerned about his own longevity, began to ply me with stories and articles about this seeming Shangri-la. On my map of Asia I finally found "Hunza" at the very northern apex of West Pakistan, flanked on the west by Afghanistan and to the east by Sinkiang Province of China. I read what books and literature I could find about the diminutive ancient kingdom hidden from the world among the towering peaks of the Karakoram Mountains, the westward extension of the better-known Himalaya Range. Some accounts by travelers, who had spent a year or more living among the natives in the valley comprising the small habitable area of this mountain kingdom, painted a prosaic picture of the inhabitants and the hard life they live—while other accounts by transient tourists described in highly romanticized superlatives the marvels of the hardy, handsome, stalwart, peace-loving, honest, friendly, noble, joyful, healthy, long-lived Hunzakuts.

I was intrigued by the legend; how it originated and how it was sustained. One of the earliest accounts of the land and peoples of Hunza was by Major John Biddulph in his book, *Tribes of the Hindoo-Koosh,* published in 1880. In it he describes the extreme isolation of the natives in their mountain stronghold, and he comments on the adverse effects of such isolation and the resulting intermarriages on the genetic stock of the Hunzakuts. "Continued intermarriage for many generations within a circumscribed area has had a most pernicious and deteriorative effect on the population," Biddulph concluded. More recent travelers have been more charitable in their assessment of the health and longevity of the natives, despite an absence of written records to document ages. One booster, early in the present century, was Sir Robert McCarrison, a highly regarded British authority on nutrition and public health. Dr. McCarrison, who spent seven years as a British army surgeon in India, noted the hardiness and good health of the Hunzakuts. He remarked on the rapidity with which they healed their wounds or infections, which he attributed largely to their diet. Later in his career, as an experimental nutritionist, he found that his white laboratory rats raised on a typical Hunzakut diet lived longer and were healthier than rats raised on the typical diets of other ethnic groups. His lectures and writings on the subject received prompt and widespread attention in the Western world. Subsequent travelers sufficiently hardy or persistent to surmount both the red tape of governmental permission and the craggy peaks of the Karakoram Mountains have done much to romanticize life, health, and longevity in Hunza.

With my interest and curiosity well kindled by the glowing descriptions I had read, I had made several attempts to obtain permission through the Pakistani Embassy in Washington to take a team of American and Pakistani physicians to Hunza for an investigation of health conditions and the local environment. Although A. Hilaly, the ambassador, had been most cordial and understanding, the response of his government to my request was an invariable "No!" This response was not altogether surprising, considering the politically "hot" location of that diminutive state at the very tip of West Pakistan, bordering on China and Afghanistan, with Russia only twelve miles away. Since Pakistan was on friendly terms with Red China it would have appeared an inhospitable act—even a hostile one—to their Red Chinese allies to allow a group of Americans to clamber over the rocks on that potentially strategic border.

Thus it was with more than casual interest that I awaited the response from Islamabad to the request by the National Geographic Society for permission to visit Hunza. After staying in Boston for almost two weeks during the start of a sabbatical from Harvard University and the Massachusetts General Hospital, I gave up waiting and flew to Oxford to commence my sabbatical year. Since the visit to Hunza was a requirement in the contract with *National Geographic,* it seemed that my adventures were over before they had begun. No sooner had I arrived in Oxford, however, than John Launois called from a phone booth in New York, informing me that permission to visit Hunza had been received. Two days later, after bidding my colleagues in Oxford good-bye in the same breath with which I had introduced myself, I met John Launois in London and our travels started.

We learned quickly that the conditions of our permission to visit Hunza were somewhat restrictive. On arriving in Karachi we were informed that we could stay in Hunza only ten days and that all our film must be turned over to Pakistani officials who would have it developed and censored before returning it to us. We also met our official guide-cum-caretaker, Aklaq Syed, who was to accompany us—and who proved indispensable not only as a translator, but also in smoothing out many situations which were to arise during our information gathering and photography.

The trip from Rawalpindi to Hunza took place in two stages: 'Pindi to Gilgit by plane and Gilgit to Hunza by jeep and foot. Both revealed the incredible scenery of the Karakoram Mountains. The twin-engine *Friendship* plane made the trip from 'Pindi to Gilgit in an hour. We flew at 17,000 feet, but even at this altitude we were among the peaks rather than above them. As far as the eye could see in all directions, the massive brown craggy mountains rose as though some supergiant had plowed this portion of the globe throwing up the earth's crust in random mounds, as his team chose an erratic course. There was some snow, but not as much as the height of the hills would seem to indicate. As it was the end of the summer, snow had largely melted on the mountains and, since precipitation is very sparse, little snow remained to be seen. As we flew past Nanga Parbit, which is approximately 27,000 feet and the fifth tallest mountain in the world, we had to crane our necks to see the top. Even Nanga Parbit seemed mostly barren of snow, so I was shocked when I learned its height. On clear days with good visibility, we were told, one can also see K-2, the second highest mountain in the world, in the distance.

Landing in Gilgit was easy after some initial apprehension. The plane came in low, headed straight at a rock wall. At the last moment a sharp swerve to the left, and we were on the runway.

Gilgit has all the hustle and bustle of a frontier town, as indeed it is. The tributaries of the Gilgit River produced the valleys of Punyal, Skardu, Yessin, Hunza, and others. Tradesmen and travelers to those valleys must pass through Gilgit to reach the outside world. Gilgit is colorful, as it is the central trading post for the frontier. Cloth, clothes, leather, and silver handicrafts seemed major items of commerce. The silver craftsmanship was especially interesting to observe, as the work is done on open charcoal fires complete with bellows right in the front of the small shops. Although much of the work is delicate filigree, the finished pieces have a rather ponderous appearance and are priced according to their equivalent weight in silver coins. Clothing shops displayed, not only silk brocades from China (reminding one that Gilgit was on the ancient silk route opened by Marco Polo), but second-hand military uniforms from many nations, and even a pre-war German train brakeman's uniform. The shops looked like the Goodwill Industries of 1930!

Our mini-caravan of two jeeps left Gilgit early on September 18, 1971. The driver and I, with luggage, occupied one jeep, and Launois, Syed, and the second driver the other. The road winds precariously along the gray and brown cliffs which form the gorge of the Hunza River. The river banks are sheer stone walls into the side of which has been scratched the narrow trail, barely wide enough to accommodate one jeep. To ride on the outside was indeed exciting. Looking down, one usually saw no road past the outer edge of the jeep but only the gray swirling waters of Hunza River a few hundred or thousand feet directly below. In some places the stone cliffs had not been indented to make the path but, rather, a ledge had been created by placing one rock in a chink in the side of the cliff, placing another flat stone atop that and continuing this process until a jutting ledge had been created. No cement held the stones together, and, needless to say, periodically such ledges collapsed into the river below. The Hunzakuts joked that their drivers are all perfect: one slip and one was no longer a driver. The Mir, hereditary ruler of the State of Hunza, told us later that he loses several drivers and jeeps each year on the road.

After passing the narrow portion of the road, the gorge broadens and the road is wider. But now it passes through loose shale which intermittently, but frequently, slides down the mountainside to cover the road. We drove as far as the town of Hindi, where we learned that the road ahead was blocked by slides and blasting. The last ten or so miles to Hunza we hiked, passing evidence of road construction on all sides; tractors from Ohio, Japan, and Russia in various stages of repair were strewn along the route. The Pakistani Army Corps of Engineers was doing the road construction, working in shifts around the clock. We, of course, could not understand the reason for such feverish activity in this remote locale. When we inquired, we were told that a Chinese trade delegation was expected to visit Gilgit in a week, and the Pakistanis were attempting to improve the route as a gesture of welcome. Actually, it was only a month after we left Hunza that the fighting between Pakistan and India broke out (in November 1971), and we then understood the urgency of opening up the Karakoram Highway. As this was the road connecting China with Pakistan, it would be the route by which supplies and personnel could be sent, if necessary, from China to aid Pakistan. This explained the prohibition of our photographing the road construction and the strict limitations imposed upon our visit to Hunza by the Pakistani ministry of defense which had seemed so irrational to us at the time. During the two weeks of our visit, however, the new road, which had been formally opened in February 1971 by Yang Chieh, Chinese communications minister, and General Abdul Hamid Khan, Pakistani army chief of staff, was not passable. The colonel in charge at Hindi gave permission for our jeeps and drivers—but not "the Americans"—to cross the bridge to the Nagar side of the Hunza River and proceed to Hunza by that alternate route while John Launois, Syed, and I hiked the remaining miles.

It was cool and pleasant at 7 A.M. that mid-September morning when we started off with one porter carrying the camera equipment. We crossed the first roadblock easily and walked slowly, photographing scenery and elderly persons walking (as we were) from Hindi to Hunza. The scenery became breathtaking as we caught our first glimpse of the snowy slopes of Rakaposhi, the peaks of which, at 25,550 feet, were to loom over us throughout our stay in Hunza. One old man clutching a live chicken to his tattered shirt kept pace with us. The chicken seemed to constitute the entirety of his worldly possessions. Unfortunately, he spoke only the local dialect, as did the others walking the road, so communication was impossible.

About 10 A.M. our progress was stopped when we arrived at a point where the Corps of Engineers were ready to dynamite the road. The explosions were louder and closer than expected. After fleeing back down the road to avoid the blast, we returned to cross the dynamited areas as soon as clearance was granted. The dust had hardly settled as we crossed, and the porter who walked ahead with the cameras narrowly missed being buried when a hail of stones fell just ahead of him. I felt most nervous as I scampered as quickly as possible over the loose rocks and sand which had completely erased the road. One glance to the right showed me the river several hundred feet directly below. With the metastable state of the hillside so soon after the blast, I was breathless and much relieved when this portion of the trail was behind us.

We hiked along and noon brought very hot sun. Heat and dust made uncomfortable traveling companions for us. We made one stop to boil water for instant coffee. Nearby natives moved in, and one brought a huge cucumber which was very juicy but not very tasty. Another offered us a plate of grapes and peaches. The fruit was remarkably delicious, better than anything we get in our stores at home, even though it looked plain and uninteresting. We were to be regaled by such delicious fruits repeatedly in Hunza.

When we came to the junction of Hyderabad River with the larger Hunza River, we could see evidence of further blasting ahead—another four to six miles across the valley, we guessed. When we crossed the Hyderabad River and arrived at the site of road construction, we dropped below the level of the road and crossed fields until we passed the area of the fault in the road. Then we had a most grueling climb back up the rocky hillside on to the road. We were relieved to find our jeeps waiting for us after the long day of rough hiking in dust and sun. It was a short drive on to Baltit and the guest house located just below the Mir's palace on the steep side of the valley. Our pleasure at the drive across the valley, with its narrow jeep trail rimmed on one side by rushing irrigation waters and on the other by an acute drop off into the valley below, competed with our eagerness to get out of our hot, sticky, dust-laden clothing.

The valley looks like one large formal garden. Surrounding hillsides are terraced and divided by stone walls like New England farms into postage-stamp-sized plots. The population is clustered into several small villages separated by the cultivated patches. The milky waters of the Hunza River with their noisy rapids seem miles below; they separate Hunza from the neighboring state of Nagar. The real drama and breathtaking beauty of the valley can be credited to the surrounding mountains. Rakaposhi at 25,550 feet looms largest across the river on the Nagar side in the direction from which we had entered the valley. Minapin, at 24,000 feet, also across the river, adds her majesty to the scene. Up the Hunza side of the valley a six-hundred-year-old fort dominates the scene, even though it is dwarfed by the towering snow-capped hills of Ulter Ber immediately behind it. I had grown up in Seattle in the shadow of Mount Ranier, but its 14,408-foot elevation would appear stunted alongside these giants. Lord Curzon, after a visit to Hunza in 1916, wrote that "the little state of Hunza alone is said to contain more summits of over 20,000 feet than there are over 10,000 feet in the entire Alps." The valley runs due east and west. North of us over other snow-covered peaks, and about forty miles away is the Chinese border across which the Mir of Hunza, great-grandfather to the present Mir, retreated when the British invaded and conquered the state almost without bloodshed in 1892. With the exception of foreign affairs, communications, and defense, the Mir has remained the absolute, but benevolent monarch in this tiny state of some 7000 square miles of mountaintops. We found the English speaking Mir to be well informed, gracious, friendly, and very helpful.

Sitting out on the terrace of the Mir's guest house, one can survey the daily activities of the Hunzakuts; a varied collection of domestic tableaus which bring to mind a Brueghel landscape. The temperature in September was balmy; cool in the morning and evening, but around 90° F. at noon. Winter brings snow and cold down into the valley. The air is dry and pleasant, but a constant fine dust is an inevitable part of the scene. The land is extremely arid, and only the ingenious irrigation system, which brings water from the glaciers and springs in the hills high above, lends greenness to the scene. The Hunzakuts are justly proud of the remarkable engineering feat that this irrigation system represents, a system which their fathers and forefathers created over a span of more than eight hundred years.

To cite an altitude for Hunza is virtually meaningless, as even the valley exists only as a steep slope. However, the Hunza River here is some 5000 to 7000 feet above sea level, and the towns of Baltit and Karimabad perhaps another 1000 to 2000 feet above the river. Hunza economy depends on its crops of wheat, barley, two or three kinds of millet, peas, broad beans, and various pulses. Vegetables grown during the summer months include cabbage, cauliflower, peas, beans, spinach, potatoes, carrots, and turnips. Tomatoes, chilies, brinjals, and gourds are dried in the summer and stocked for consumption in the winter. During the summer fresh vegetables and fruits are bountiful, but in winter, potatoes, turnips, dried vegetables, fruits (the delicious apricots and grapes), and almonds are available in limited amounts. The economy has been a bare subsistence one, and in the past the end of winter in Hunza saw hunger and privation before spring brought relief with new greens.

Although no official census has disturbed the tranquility of the valley, the Mir of Hunza states that the population of his country is 40,000, but that 15,000 of these are "down country." "With the roads the young people go to Pakistan for military service or employment. They return and change the traditional ways of my people. The diet is changing and health is deteriorating. There are fewer old people now." The Mir's authority is absolute in internal affairs of his state; he holds court each morning at 10 A.M. with his council of elders and *wazir* (vizier) and listens to and arbitrates all disputes among his countrymen. He claims there are no crimes of violence or passion, no robberies. Only when there is little snow in the mountains (causing a shortage of water for irrigation) do disputes arise over the distribution of the water. He walks freely among his subjects without guard; and the palace, as we saw, is not guarded. He says that the young people returning from "down country" represent a dissident element, but, he concluded with a smile, "Thank God we have no problems yet with the students."

Water is Hunza's most valued resource. The Hunza River contains so much silt it is almost gray. The water in the irrigation ditches which is used for all purposes—drinking, washing, bathing—is similarly opaque with a gray silt which refuses to settle. The Mir makes a point of drinking this murky water, saying that it is healthful and conducive to a long life. There is, however, clear spring water at his palace for the Rani and his guests.

The origins of the peoples of Hunza are lost in antiquity. A popular tale attributes their beginnings to three soldiers who deserted from the army of Alexander the Great, each of whom married an Indian princess and hid in the wild hills of the Karakoram. However, Professor Karl Jettmar of the South Asian Institute of the University of Heidelberg, whom we met in Gilgit during his fifth visit to this area, explained that such a mythical origin was applied to many tribes in these remote areas. He says that early Indo-Aryan tribes coming from the west and northwest across what is now Afghanistan from West Turkistan and Iran mixed with the people of the mountains. These people are non-Mongoloid and look Caucasian. Although Hunza has been on the silk route joining China with India and the west, the occasional caravans passing through since Marco Polo's time have disturbed the isolation of these people very little. "For generations the tribes of Hunza had been roving bands of robbers who lived off the caravan trade between China and India. They had to move long distances rapidly in order to surprise the caravans in ambush. For this they had to be very sturdy, and the strong and healthy survived," Professor Jettmar said.

The Hunzakuts abandoned this warlike existence in the nineteenth century, and their firearms have been used by several generations only for hunting. T. Burrow, professor of Sanskrit at Oxford University, attributes the individual character of the language to the long isolation of these mountain people. "Their language, Burashaski, resembles no other language on earth and indicates that the people of Hunza have been isolated in these mountains since the Aryan migrations about 1500 B.C." Besides the main language of Burashaski, Wakhi (an Iranian language) is spoken in the north and Shena (an Indo-Aryan language) in the south. In the village of Mommabad with a population of only two hundred, a fourth language, Bereski, is spoken.

The absence of a written language meant that no birth records were available. Furthermore, the only event in their long history of which westerners are aware was the invasion of Hunza by the British in 1892. Though we asked the old people what they remembered of this event, the unreliability of ages determined by this method must be appreciated. I will relate the ages that we were told in what follows. It was the large number of very vigorous elderly persons we encountered who managed the steep hillsides with much greater ease and agility than did we, that so impressed us. Their actual ages I cannot vouch for.

Our first day in Hunza was a full one. We slept well but the sun and long hike of the previous day had had their effects, and I was stiff, dehydrated, and sunburned. After a Western-style breakfast of oatmeal, fried eggs, plus *chappati* (unleavened flat bread) fried in oil, we got into the jeep and drove up to the fort. From the roof of the fort one can look down on all the activities of the valley. During the summer people live on the roofs of their square stone houses. Here they dry the grapes, apricots, vegetables, and grains on which they will subsist through the winter. One can spot the women easily by the bright colors of their scarves, blouses, and voluminous baggy pants. They were very shy, covering their faces and turning away as we approached, but one often caught dark furtive eyes peering inquisitively at us. For several centuries the population had been Shiite Muslim; relatively recently they have been converted to the Ismaili sect and are now followers of the Aga Khan.

A few hundred yards down the hill from the fort was Hunza's single school. We found the children on the school grounds having their drill and exercises. Our first glimpse of the youngsters, ages six to twelve, was of them marching goose step around the grounds marking time with "left-right" in English.

The schoolmaster, Sultan-Ali, age fifty, proved to be a very interesting fellow. After introductions, he addressed me, saying, "I am the humble schoolmaster here. I speak six languages: English, Urdu, Burashaski, Persian [and two tongues I'd never heard of before]. You, Professor, are a learned, highly educated person; how many languages do you speak?" I don't think my mumbled response that scientists in America generally were not very adept at languages impressed him nearly as much as his linguistic accomplishments had me. He explained that he had been trained in education in Gilgit and spent six years with the Gilgit Scouts, a crack English regiment of mountain troops which the Pakistani had preserved. The Hunza school was started by the Aga Khan as a gift to Hunza on the occasion of his diamond jubilee (he was weighed in diamonds that year!). The subjects taught were English, Mathematics, "General Knowledge" (geography and history), and Theology (Islamic). Some 350 students attended school. All males six to twelve years of age were supposed to attend school six days a week from 8:00 A.M. to 1:30 P.M. with a short day on Friday. Clearly all children in this age group were not conforming to this rule, as we could judge from the ragged spectators observing with fascination the marching and gymnastics of their more fortunate brothers. We observed one history class during which the teacher read a few words of text which was then repeated as a chant by the students. The text was about Abraham Lincoln—but in Urdu. It seemed to me that such bright-looking children deserved something better than rote learning; but at least the educational process had started in Hunza. Although we were fortunate to have the schoolmaster, Sultan-Ali, assigned as our guide by the Mir during our stay in Hunza, our visit did nothing to foster education as the school had to close down for ten days for lack of a schoolmaster.

From the school we went to visit the single (twelve-bed) hospital in the state, which I was particularly interested to see. There I spoke to Dr. Sahoor Ahmed, M.B., B.S. (Punjab). He was posted in Hunza by the Pakistani ministry of health to satisfy his two-year service requirement. He had volunteered for Hunza to see the north and had been here for eight months. He is the only doctor within forty miles—and the only one in all of Hunza and neighboring Nagar states. There are eight dispensaries and one hospital with the dispensaries staffed by nonphysicians. Dr. Ahmed estimated that there were some 40,000 persons in his catchment area, and it was his impression that the Hunzakuts were not exceptionally healthy.

Dr. Ahmed had no obstetrical practice, as men are not allowed to be present at a birth; only older women of the immediate family are permitted. Mothers nurse their offspring for two years and wean them gradually onto fruits and adult foods. Infant mortality is higher than in Punjab, Dr. Ahmed told us. Diarrheal disorders are the major cause of infant deaths. He found malnutrition, anemia, worms, goiter with many cretins, and pneumonia to be common. There was a smallpox outbreak with three or four deaths in the past year. There is no immunization program. Tuberculosis is found among the young males who go "down country" for military service and employment in Pakistan, but women also have tuberculosis. There is much bronchial asthma. He recounted the diseases he had seen during his eight months in residence as: one stroke with hemiplegia, five cases of rheumatic fever with joint involvement but no heart murmurs, one case of gonorrhea but no syphilis, two cases of hypertension, two cases of cancer (one leukemic and one rectal), no angina or heart attacks, and no kidney stones or renal disease. Everyone, he claimed, had worms— round worms, tapeworms, and threadworms. Amebic dysentery was rare. There was no alcoholism and no drug problems. Older people don't smoke, but most young people do.

The doctor showed me his pharmacy, which is stocked by the government, and his surgical unit which seemed quite busy, but mostly with minor cuts and injuries. He did no major surgery and very few fractures occurred. When I asked to see the hospital he took me in back of the dispensary to show me two small single-story buildings: one for women, the other for men. Both were empty. The last male patient had asthma, I was told, and had been discharged ten days earlier; the last female patient was also an asthmatic and had left the hospital eight days earlier. This seemed strange for a population of 40,000—either the population was remarkably healthy or they were grossly underutilizing their single medical facility because of mistrust or cultural incompatabilities with Western medical practices.

At the hospital we met Kabul Hyat, age ninety-nine, who had been the bodyguard to the previous Mir when the British had invaded. He proved to be the village clown, full of stories that had everyone laughing. He described three generations of his offspring. He was lively, and, though we couldn't understand his words, his vivid gestures, the merry twinkle in his eyes, and his infectious humor had us laughing together with the small crowd who gathered about him. He told how there are four species of ducks in Hunza. One rare species has curled tail feathers, just like his moustache. The other Hunzakuts don't have a moustache like his, he joked, because they didn't know about this rare duck—Kabul's moustache was coal black and curled up at the ends. The next day he proudly danced for us showing no signs of physical infirmity. Later the Mir confirmed Kabul's story of having served as his grandfather's bodyguard in 1892.

That evening we had dinner with the Mir. We signed the royal guest book and noted that, though the first entry was dated 1917, the list of visitors had fewer than one hundred names. After dinner the Mir related bits of historical background. Apparently the agreement with the Pakistani government regarding defense, foreign affairs, and communications is identical to that Hunza had with the British prior to partition in 1947 when Hunza was part of Kashmir. The British held a plebiscite to determine the fate of Kashmir during the partition. Despite the fact that the populace was overwhelmingly Moslem, the Maharaja of Kashmir joined India, even though the Mir had warned him that Hunza, with its Ismaili religion, would revolt. They did revolt, broke off relations with the Maharaja, and joined Pakistan.

The first jeep arrived in Hunza in 1948 and that event brought the Age of the Jeep. Together with the new road the jeep is revolutionizing Hunza through contact with the outside world. Although a bicycle had been brought in before the jeep as the first form of wheeled transportation, it must have been totally useless with the steep terrain and loose sand of the narrow paths. Already the self-reliant and totally independent Hunzakuts were becoming accustomed to goods and food brought in by jeep. In the past the clothes they wore had all been made from the cloth they wove of the wool from their own sheep, but now they are dressed in brightly colored cotton prints from Japan. Imported tea is replacing the traditional drinks of fruit juice. Small shops are appearing in the villages as natives turn to commerce rather than agriculture for their livelihood. The old people told us repeatedly, that "Life is much easier and goods are plentiful now, but no one has time for relaxation and festivities any more!" The Mir claims that the health of his people is deteriorating.

There now is minimal electrification in the valley. When the first president of Pakistan spent five days relaxing and hunting as the guest of the Mir, he asked the Mir what he might do for Hunza. The Mir asked him to help them obtain hydroelectric power. President Ayub Khan arranged a grant for 700,000 rupees (about $64,000), and in 1969 the lights went on in Hunza.

Once our interest in the old people became known, they began to visit us. Thus we met Ghalum Mohammed Shah, age 100, waiting for us at the guest house when we returned one evening. He was twenty or twenty-one at the time of the British invasion of Hunza in 1892, he told us. He appeared lean and agile and still works breaking rocks for the road. He showed us the iron sledgehammer which he uses. I estimated its weight at about five pounds, but he flourished it with ease with one hand. He had had seven sons by his first wife, but she and all sons were now deceased. His second wife gave birth to three sons and four daughters. Some had died in infancy and two in their teens due to an infectious disease characterized by boils. He told us that there were many more old people when he was a child than there are now. His tan face was rimmed with a gray beard. He wore the typical white woolen pancake hat with rolled brim that can be pulled down over the ears during the cold. A worn brown army shirt and light pajamalike cotton trousers, comprised his attire. He wielded his hammer deftly as he showed us how he shaped stones to build a wall. His pulse was regular at seventy-six beats per minute. His blood pressure was normal at 145 systolic and 88 diastolic. There were no heart murmurs and his peripheral arteries were soft. He was without teeth, and the only other abnormality I discerned was a small goiter which we noted commonly in this iodine-poor area.

Coming up the hill from our guest house we were overtaken by three elders who walked up the twenty- or thirty-degree incline without pause or difficulty while we stopped every few steps to catch our breath and quiet our pounding hearts. The oldest of the two was Ali Murad, age ninety-one, whose prominent red hair and beard (henna stained) we had admired as he danced at celebrations the previous day, marking the wedding of the crown prince of Hunza. Murad, like the other two, was a member of the Mir's council of elders. He is a farmer and still does a little work on the land. He has five living children and had three who have died. He claimed to be about eight years old at the time of the British invasion in 1892, which would have made him eighty-eight rather than ninety-one years old. He attributes his longevity to the local food, much walking, hard work, and Hunza water. The term for Hunza water is *"Hunza panna,"* but this is also the name for the raw red wine so much prized by the Hunzakuts. Thus, whether Murad was referring to the murky, silt-laden water or the fresh red wine I'll never know. The second male was Ali Shah, age eighty-nine years, also a farmer. He calls his vigor and health "God given." The third elder was Shah Malik, age eighty, a farmer.

The high social status of the elderly in Hunza was typified by two aspects of their culture. The oldest individuals from each of the little villages gathered every morning at the palace of the Mir. While the latter presided, the elders—sitting on rugs on the floor in a semicircle before him—listened to and arbitrated disputes and established the rules which governed the little state. The old people were clearly respected for their wisdom. By being continually challenged in this manner by younger colleagues they retained their mental faculties. The impetus to preserve mental faculties through continued use, I believe, is very important psychologically for the elderly.

The cultural life of Hunza calls for frequent festivities, and since we had the good fortunate of visiting at the time of the wedding of the crown prince we saw much of their traditional celebration. Dancing plays an important part in all Hunza festivities. We joined a crowd gathered in a large rectangle in a field. In the periphery were the musicians: two marching drums, two small hemispheric drums, and three reeds resembling oboes. The music was very rhythmic, with the oboes maintaining a constant flurry of nasal whining notes. To this rhythmical noise men were dancing. From two to six or more men stand at the start of each piece and solemnly go through a series of foot-stamping movements, which are not intricate and are accompanied by minimal body and arm movements. The first dancer in the line sets the action and the movements of the others diminish progressively to the last dancer. Invariably it was the oldest man who led the dance, another indication of their high social status. We watched our ninety-nine-year-old clowning, moustachioed friend, Kabul, lead the dancers. Occasionally a dance was livened by a sequence of hopping on one foot and then on the other, but this was generally short lived. The dancers moved gradually around a circle within a ring of male spectators. Women do not participate in such activities—or, in fact, in any aspect of the social life—but their bright-colored garments could be seen in the house tops and among nearby trees as they clandestinely observed the antics of their menfolk. The music was so exotic to my ear that the musicians could have been repeating the same piece all day. Actually, the musicians performed about eight hours that day. The Mir informed us that the musicians came from a separate sect which produces only musicians and blacksmiths! Colorful as the dancing was, it soon became tedious in its ponderous repetitiousness, and I felt it could have benefited greatly by some female participation; but it did again emphasize the important role of the elderly in the culture of Hunza.

As part of the traditional royal wedding festivities the Mir is obliged to feed his subjects. Toward this end about ten yaks were brought down from their pasture land in the high Pamirs across the Chinese border where the mirs of Hunza have held hereditary pastures. For several days prior to the feast these remarkable, huge, black, buffalolike beasts grazed peaceably on the Mir's lawn. They were finally barbecued and served up to the gathered populace, each of whom were entitled to a morsel of the Mir's bounty.

We were only privileged to see and photograph an elderly woman after we had been in Hunza several days. The Moslem religion keeps the womenfolk well protected from contact with male strangers. Only in 1959 did the present Rani make unveiled appearances at social gatherings in her home. Begum Murad Shah, age ninety, graciously invited us into her home to take pictures. She has five children, all of whom were living, and two grandchildren. She married at age nineteen, and her husband is also ninety. Neither remembered the arrival of the British. She attributes her longevity to the good climate, the water, and the wonderful fruit, which is eaten fresh during the summer and dried during the winter.

The oldest inhabitant of the valley, we were told, was Tulah Beg, age 110, who remembered the arrival of the British when he was about twenty-six years old. We watched him climb the steep path slowly, invariably aided by a staff. He doesn't work any more. My superficial examination revealed him to be a feeble elderly male with a large painless or indolent skin cancer on his forehead. His peripheral pulses were easily felt and his arteries soft, indicative of little arteriosclerosis. His blood pressure was normal (152/84) and his pulse 90 and regular. His lungs were clear. His reflexes were active and symmetrical in both arms and legs. He had no edema—no excess of body fluid. Though he was very thin and somewhat feeble, his weathered features, erect posture, and bushy henna-stained beard gave him the appearance of a biblical patriarch. He was accompanied by his two sons, Nigar Shah, age seventy-four, and Sagi Ali, age seventy, both very vigorous. One son served as our porter, shouldering a heavy box of John Launois's photographic equipment and bounding with it over the forbidding terrain "like an agile mountain goat."

We passed a delightful old man, age ninety-five, Gul Baig, from the nearby village of Aliabad. He had a jaunty step, swinging his arms, and an upright bearing. He had smooth tanned facial skin and a henna-stained beard. When I asked him why he dyed his beard, he replied, "To give joy." Then he insisted that we come to his home while he demonstrated the process for us. First he dropped a marble-sized crystal of rock salt into an ounce of water and stirred for a minute. When the crystal was removed, a handful of ground henna powder was stirred into the water to produce a mustardlike paste with a grayish-green color. This mess he then applied to his beard and worked it in well with his finger tips. He covered his beard with a piece of plastic wrapping and then with a dirty cloth, which he bound over his chin like a surgical mask. After thirty minutes to "bind" the dye, he removed the mask and the excess henna he washed off with water amid much sputtering and spitting. This dyeing was done at two-week intervals.

Having examined his face closely as I observed the dyeing I noticed he wore black eye makeup. I learned that Hunzakuts blacken their eyelids with a stick of what looks like graphite and lead. This is rubbed in a groove in a block of similar material and the stick then applied to the eyelid and actually introduced within the conjunctival sac. With a final flourish Gul Baig drew a black line laterally at the corner of his eye as an actor's eye makeup (or my daughter's!). This treatment is supposed to protect against the many eye infections which are so prevalent. Many of the small children had black eye makeup, too, but I didn't discover whether this was for medicinal or cosmetic purposes.

Such in brief is the modern state of Hunza—but it is changing rapidly. Long after leaving it, I still ponder whether health and longevity in Hunza were fact or myth. Surely the very breathtaking setting of this mini-state, dwarfed beneath the towering majesty of its surrounding peaks, elicits the poet in the observer; and it is easy to transfer to the natives the serenity and timelessness of the setting.

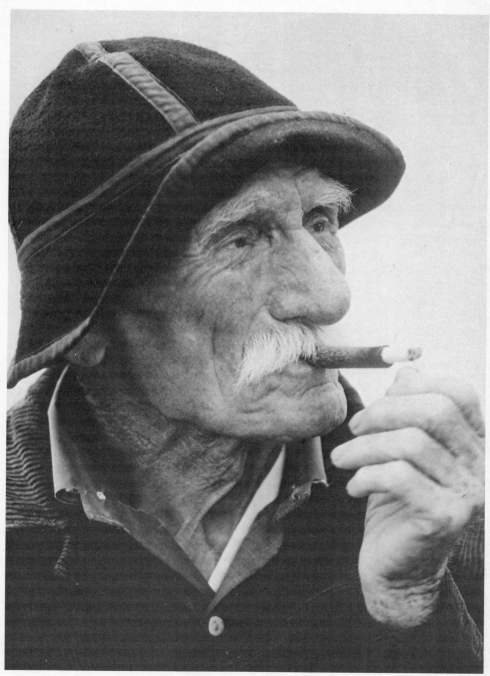

113-year-old Chu Khasheeg enjoys a cigar.

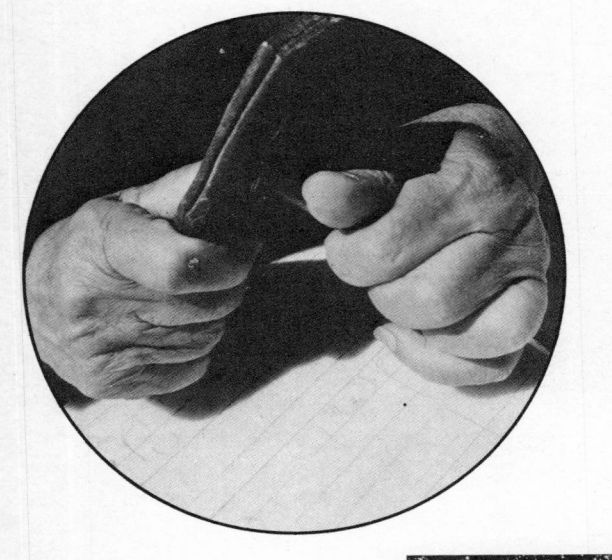

The hands of Roman Ytmeledzhe, age ninety. He is engraving a tombstone, a craft that he has followed since childhood.

Ninety-five-year-old Mikhail Mchedleshvili chopping wood. He frequently engages in such activities.

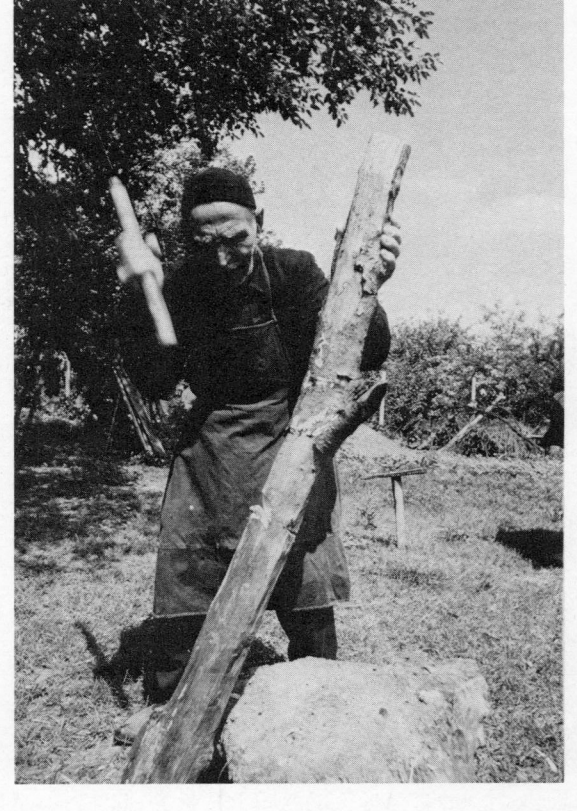

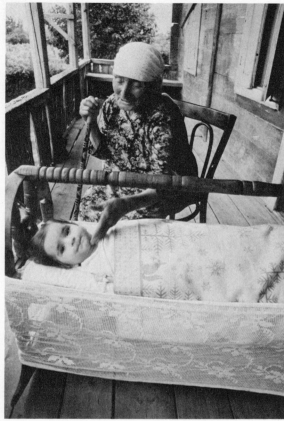

Khfaf Lasuria, who is probably 130 years old, sits beside the cradle of her great-great-granddaughter.

Khfaf Lasuria takes a drink of wine.

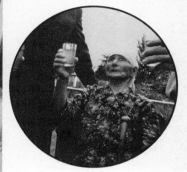

Khedzhgva Sukhba, 105 years old, watering flowers on the grave of her son.

Ninety-nine-year-old Anna Gurgenishvili hoes in her garden.

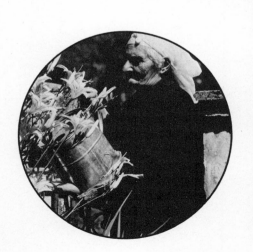

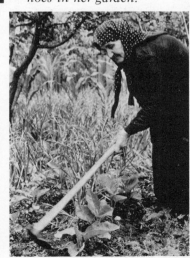

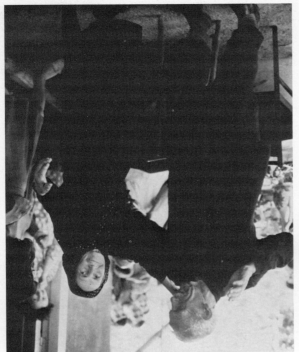

Karum Utiashvili, ninety-five, embraces his wife, Keke, who is eighty years old.

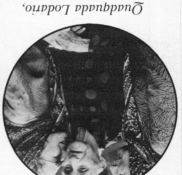

Quaquada Lodario, 108, listens to her friends, Simitsia and Nina Aridzba, ninety and ninety-three.

Karum Utiashvili dances with his wife, Keke.

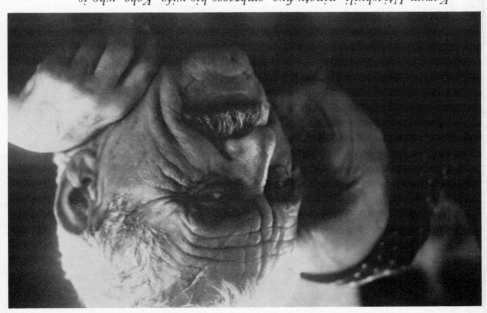

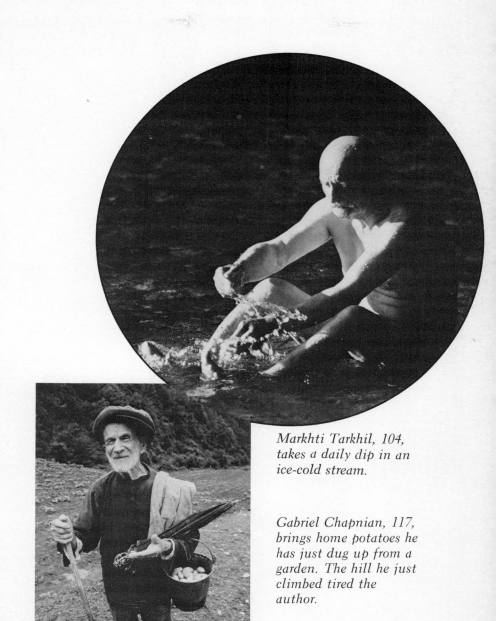

Markhti Tarkhil, 104, takes a daily dip in an ice-cold stream.

Gabriel Chapnian, 117, brings home potatoes he has just dug up from a garden. The hill he just climbed tired the author.

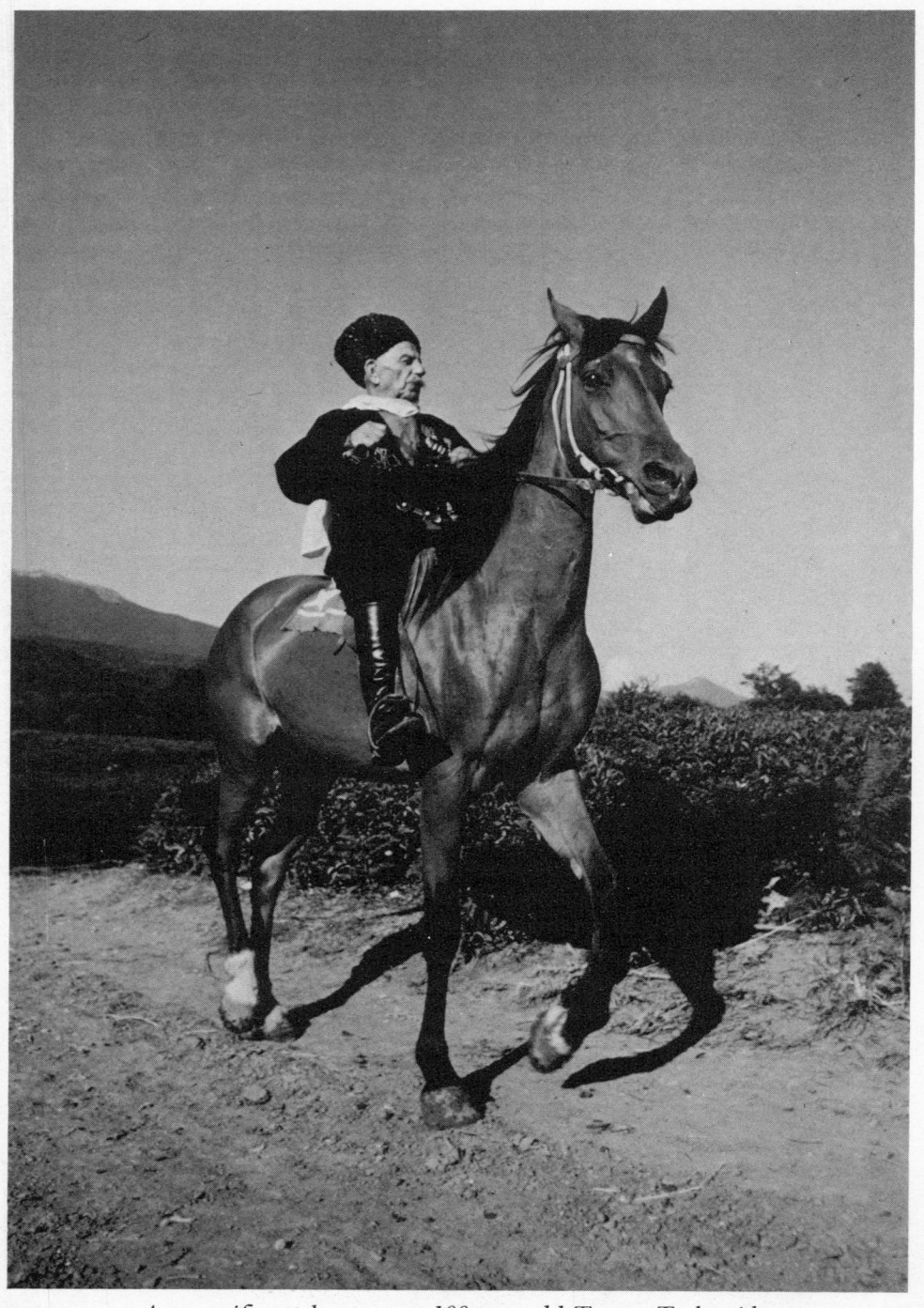

A magnificent horseman, 100-year-old Temur Tarba rides through a tea plantation.

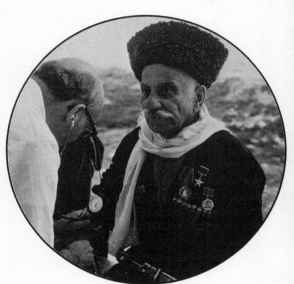

The author examines Temur Tarba, who is wearing some of his medals, among them the prized "Hero of Labor" award.

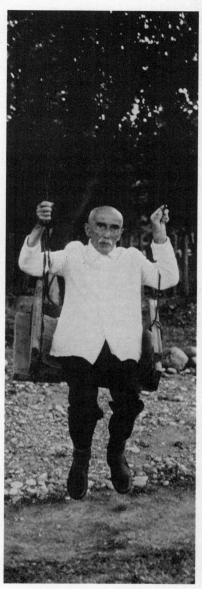

Ninety-six-year-old Shukri Agrba is enjoying a swing in his village of Eshery.

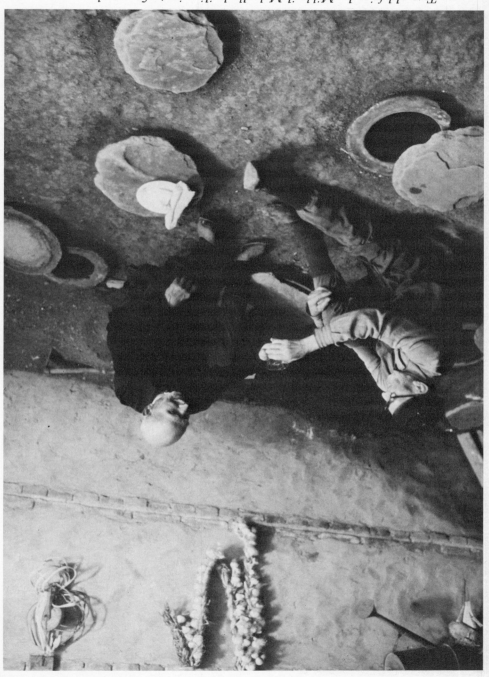

Two old friends, Mikhail Mchedleshvili, ninety-five, and Gyorgi Gvelykashvili, eighty-seven, enjoy a sip of homemade Georgian wine. Each ceramic vat in the floor holds 40 gallons.

3

VILCABAMBA

No wise man ever wished to be younger.

Jonathan Swift (1667–1745), *Thoughts on Various Subjects, Moral and Diverting*

As in the case of Hunza and the Caucasus, one can find, on searching into the past, references to unusual health and longevity in this region. One such account is recorded in *Voyages to Various Parts of the World,* which is the journal of Captain George Coggeshall, dated June 1825. Captain Coggeshall remarks on the "pure air and healthful location . . . [near Payta, Peru, close to Vilcabamba, where] many of its inhabitants live to a very great age. While I was here, a man died who was said to be 111 years old. I went . . . from curiosity, to see several old people, that were from 90 to 100 years. Among others we visited an old man and his wife, the latter was 100 years of age, and the husband probably somewhat older. He appeared to retain his mental faculties, and was able to walk about. . . . They live extremely simple, retire to rest at nightfall, and rise at daylight."

Much more recently an American physician, Dr. Eugene Paine, who spent twenty-five years studying diseases in South America, wrote in the *Reader's Digest* of November 1954 that the province in which Vilcabamba is situated was remarkably free of heart disease. In 1959 another American, Albert Kramer, came to Vilcabamba and was "cured" of heart disease by living there, according to his account. He also stated that the inhabitants of the area showed remarkable longevity as well as freedom from heart disease.

In 1969 high governmental officials in Ecuador requested Dr. Miguel Salvador, a prominent cardiologist of Quito, to investigate the rumors about unusual longevity and health in Vilcabamba. Dr. Salvador accepted the assignment with considerable reservations because of doubts of his own about the rumors. Nevertheless, he organized a team of physicians and technicians which met in Vilcabamba in March 1969, where they made observations on thirty-eight percent of the population. A further study was conducted by Dr. Salvador a year later and the information he has collected and published constitutes the factual basis for including Vilcabamba in this account.

In September 1970, on my way to Vilcabamba, I flew to Quito with my colleague, Dr. Harold Elrick, to meet Dr. Salvador. Dr.

Elrick's brother, Earle M. Elrick, encouraged and generously supported our little expedition. Dr. Salvador graciously made available the data from his two studies, which provided excellent background material for our visit. He also made arrangements with the appropriate officials in Vilcabamba so that our stay was highly efficient and our welcome there was a warm one. After investigating the possible flights we made a quick decision to rent a car and drive from Quito to Vilcabamba down the Pan-American Highway which runs along the Andes, the backbone of Ecuador. Most of the route is a single-lane, rutted dirt road passing along the steep side of mountains, over high passes and through beautiful green valleys. The road was occasionally crossed by other country lanes, but we navigated by compass, always choosing the southern course whenever a question of the correct route arose. The roughness of the road took its toll on the car. One especially cold and windy day the draft seemed particularly disagreeable. I rolled up my window, and my companion did likewise; but the draft persisted. Looking around we noted that the back end of the car—including the rear window—had fallen off. When we returned the car to the agency in Quito, they just couldn't believe we had not been in a wreck with it. They didn't appreciate the power of their own rural roads. It is the only time I have gotten the better of a car rental agency! Nevertheless, the trip was enjoyable and instructive; the air was crisp, cool, sunny, and invigorating at altitudes between 5000 and 10,000 feet. We had numerous opportunities to observe and speak with the inhabitants in towns and in the countryside so that when we arrived in Loja we did not feel like total strangers.

In Loja, a city of 25,000 inhabitants and the capital of the province in which Vilcabamba lies, we were greeted graciously by the prefect, who afforded us every assistance. The ride to Vilcabamba was only twenty-five miles farther but took nearly three hours and would not have been possible without the jeep and driver put at our disposal by the prefect. Thus, Vilcabamba shares to a small degree the features of remoteness and isolation which characterize Hunza.

Vilcabamba, which in the language of the Inca Indians means "Sacred Valley," is in a valley of the Andes at an altitude of some 4500 feet, not far from the Peruvian border and about 100 miles inland from the Pacific Ocean. It enjoys a very even, comfortable climate with an average year-round temperature of 68° F. and almost no seasonal variation. In every way it seemed a typical, small, rural agricultural community, with unpaved streets and adobe houses, dominated by an old church across from the village square. However, a census taken at our request and with the support of Dr. Salvador in 1971 by the Instituto Nacional de Estatistica of Ecuador recorded a total population of 819, with nine individuals over the age of 100 years. This is, of course, too small a population base upon which to make a valid comparison on a national scale. However, the normalized figure of 1100 centenarians per 100,000 of population for Vilcabamba contrasts with figures of 63 per 100,000 of population in Azerbaijan, thirty-nine for Georgia, and three for the United States does emphasize the unusually high proportion of centenarians in this small community. The percent of inhabitants in this small village over sixty years of age is 11.4, as contrasted with 4.5 percent for rural Ecuador generally. Furthermore, there is very little movement of populations in this area; we are not dealing with a Palm Springs or Miami Beach where many old people migrate late in life.

Dr. Salvador has affirmed that the number of nine centenarians is correct for the time of the census. However, the number may not be truly accurate, he relates, since some of the people leave the village to hide from public officials, thinking that the census is to obtain more taxes for the government. In his first visit to Vilcabamba in 1969, Dr. Salvador claims to have found thirteen persons over 100 years old, but on his return the next year he could no longer find that many; some had either stayed away or had died.

We found Vilcabamba to be quite inaccessible. Although it is only some twenty-five miles from Loja, this distance is covered by an unpaved, single-lane, rutted road which winds through the hilly Andes generally following narrow valleys with switchbacks between cultivated fields clinging to the steep green hillside. One requires four-wheel drive—and three hours—to negotiate the rough journey. Streams and river beds must be crossed and steep mountain slopes climbed. With torrential rains not infrequently blocking the road to Loja, all traffic—a rare bus and a few jeeps—is stopped until bulldozers scrape out a new road. When this occurs few people in the Vilcabamba region hear about it—only those who wait patiently for the rare bus to take them with their bananas or few chickens to sell for a bit of cash in Loja.

A small church across from an unkempt square crowded with a

tangle of flowering bushes provides the focus for the community. Unpaved streets are lined by adobe huts, with pigs, chickens, and children providing the major traffic. Hygienic and public health considerations have little impact on life in Vilcabamba. Pigs scavenge on the earthen floor and chickens roost on the table while the family has a meal. The Chamba and Vilcabamba rivers touch the edge of the village and provide water for drinking, bathing, and washing. Bathing is an infrequent event; many old people reporting a bath only once in two years—and the longest interval claimed was ten years! Much of life is spent out of doors, as the one- to two-room huts accommodate six persons on the average and ten or more in many instances. Only one-tenth of the population has access to sanitary facilities; only eighteen percent of the habitations have electricity. Farming engages sixty percent of the working population and major crops include corn, yucca, coffee, tobacco, bananas, potatoes, oats, wheat, sugarcane, grapes, barley, beans, and peanuts. Age-old farming methods are utilized, and long hours of heavy labor are required to obtain a livelihood despite the seeming natural lushness of the valley. The population is of mixed Indian and Spanish extraction with distinctly European features predominant in the elderly citizens. On a return visit in 1974 blood samples were taken and determination of blood groups revealed that even the older individuals whom we had thought from their appearance might be purely European stock had considerable admixture with native Indians.

Catholicism is the religion of nearly all the citizens. We found the old people, especially the women, to be quite devout. The baptismal records helped us in establishing the ages of the old people, but this did not prove as simple as it might sound. Not all the old people were included in the baptismal records which are extant, and we had to check carefully that the birth listed in the baptismal records was actually that of the old person we knew. Two examples will suffice to illustrate the types of problems we encountered.

For Vilcabamba's alleged oldest citizen, Miguel Carpio, and his neighboring cousin, Gabriel Erazo, no baptismal records were available. In 1970 both claimed to be 121 years old. One of Miguel's daughters had a baptismal record that puts her age at eighty-six, and we were told that several neighbors whose advanced ages were documented remember Carpio to be an older man when they were young. Dr. Salvador thought from his own cross-checking that the stated ages of both men were credible, "yet we have no absolute proof," he added. On a recent visit I spent more time examining the baptismal records and found information on a José Miguel Carpio, who was a younger sibling of Miguel Carpio. The parents of this José Miguel Carpio were identical in name with the parents of Miguel Carpio, and from independent information from Miguel and a living brother we had confirmed that José Miguel Carpio was, in fact, the fifth younger sibling of Miguel Carpio. The baptismal record documents that José was born in 1874. Allowing approximately two years per sibling, this would make Miguel's real age some 110 years now rather than the ages of 121 claimed four years ago or the present claim of 132. One hundred ten years is surely a venerable old age but one within the documented life span of man. There is obviously a real tendency to exaggerate ages, and this apparently has increased recently with the interest of the local government and the outside world in the longevity attributed to the inhabitants of this remote valley. Recently captions have appeared under photographs of José David Toledo in the international press claiming him to be 141 years old when his stated age to us in 1970 was 107 years. We were saddened to learn on our 1974 visit that this spry elderly man, who had entertained us with his lively conversation, had died between our two visits.

Micaela Quezada's case is another which typifies the difficulties we had with age determination. We had seen her baptismal record prominently underscored by local officials in the book of birth records. She was born in 1870, according to these records. When we called on her at her home we found her sitting on her front porch. She is a placid, wrinkled, toothless elderly woman with a very sweet laugh. She is one of the few spinsters in Vilcabamba and proud of her state. Micaela claimed to be 106, which seemed in fair agreement with the documented age of 104 indicated by the baptismal record. However, on checking we found her father to be Benino Quezada and her mother Mariá de los Angeles Mendietta, and the names of her parents were confirmed by a cousin, Serafin Quezada, who lives with her and was sixty-five years old and very talkative. A return visit to the baptismal records revealed that the Micaela Quezada listed there as born in 1870 had a father named Juan Quezada and a mother named Maria Mercedes Patino. This revelation was quite disconcerting to us, as clearly the entry in the baptismal record was of a person with different parents from our living Micaela Quezada. When confronted directly by these facts Señorita Quezada said, "Oh yes, of course, that's my cousin who lived in San Pedro [a village some three miles away]. She was older than me and died some thirty or forty years ago." Thus we had been misled by accepting a baptismal record which our Ecuadorian friends had mistaken for that of the living Micaela Quezada. I was reassured again that one can resolve the baptismal records and relate them to appropriate individuals only if one knows the correct parents of the living persons.

Certainly a much more careful examination of the baptismal records is required. On our recent visit we made photographs of the first book of records. Unfortunately, the first seven pages of the book were torn out. Thus this book which started on June 17, 1852, had as its first entry after the missing seven pages birth number 54 of 1863. Much of the material is very difficult to decipher. Though it is inscribed with a clear handwriting, the heavy black ink penetrated through the page obscuring the writing on the opposite side. Such experiences as these with Miguel Carpio and Micaela Quezada made us much more cautious in accepting stated ages. It will take a zealous and persistent genealogist to sort out all the facts of interrelationships and ages in Vilcabamba. For our purposes there exists a considerable number of active oldsters whose life styles we were eager to examine. The phenomenon seemed the more unique and interesting in that it occurs in a setting of poor sanitation with very high infant mortality and malnutrition.

In the village we met some memorable characters. When we called on 110-year-old Miguel Carpio, Vilcabamba's eldest citizen, he was about to go to the barber shop for his bimonthly haircut. We inquired if we could photograph him while having his hair cut and beard trimmed, and he smilingly obliged. He was proud that his beard was still growing at his age and explained that he enjoyed his trips to the barber shop. Miguel's house is located some 100 yards from the barber, who conducts his trade on a chair out on the porch.

We talked to Uzelvira Carpio, the daughter who cares for the old man, and learned that there are 160 relatives in the Carpio family. When we inquired about a possible family reunion, she threw up her hands and said rapidly, "Impossible! Impossible! Impossible!" She then explained that few of the relatives were in Vilcabamba; they were scattered all over Ecuador.

When asked the secret of his long and active life Miguel Carpio answered, "I have been a hunter of wild animals here and elsewhere. To reach my game I had to climb up and down all the time and when I finally killed an animal I always washed in its blood. In fact, I regularly washed in animal blood most of my life, or at least until I stopped hunting around the age of seventy-five." I learned that it was common around this region to wash sick children in animal blood "to make them well." Miguel smokes and drinks, and his daughter says he still likes to flirt with the girls.

Asked if he would like to turn back the clock, Miguel thought for a long while and replied, "I would not wish to be fifteen again, but if I could take off fifteen years from my age that would be wonderful. Fifteen years ago I was in better condition than I am now. My eyesight was fine and I felt good." He was then over ninety-five years old! His diet, like that of the others, consists of grains, vegetables, fruits and a little meat.

Asked about the youth of Vilcabamba, Miguel replied, "Youth has too much freedom." Then he added, "It is the girls who chase the boys nowadays. . . . I don't understand."

On our return visit in 1974 Miguel—now 110—had aged considerably. He now moved about slowly with the aid of a cane. He complained of rheumatism and seemed quite feeble. He still enjoyed talking, however, and he cooperated cheerfully in providing blood samples and a skin biopsy.

We watched Señora Clodovea Herrera, 103, thread a needle for sewing. As were all of the elderly we saw, she was born in Vilcabamba. She was the mother of eight children, "but they are all gone now." When asked the secret of her long and healthy life, she said, "God." Her diet is also vegetables and fruits with meat once a month, "because I can't afford it more often." The most important event in her life she remembers was her first communion. Like most inhabitants of Vilcabamba she is Catholic and very pious. Her first communion took place there at the church ninety-two years ago.

When asked her impression of the moon landings, Señora Herrera reacted with a hurt expression and emphatically said, "Only God with his great power can reach the moon." Watching her response, I felt as though I had asked a sacrilegious question and I retreated.

In the local bakery we found Señora Hermelinda León, ninety-five, busily transferring freshly baked rolls from the large earthen oven to wicker baskets. She works there a couple of days each week to earn a little money, and on the remaining days she can be found from first light until dusk in her garden cultivating beans, vegetables, and bananas, which provide the staples of her diet; once a week she buys a small piece of meat.

Señora León was born in the region of Vilcabamba. She married at the age of seventeen or eighteen and had two sons and three daughters. Both sons died in infancy and only a daughter who lives in Quito survives. Her husband died thirty-seven years ago at the age of seventy. She does not own a clock and asks, "Why would I need one?" She has never seen television, although she has heard a radio, and she scoffs at reports of men on the moon.

Her health through her long life has been excellent. Until Dr. Salvador's team came to Vilcabamba she had never seen a doctor. When they left they told her she had a good heart and was in excellent condition. When questioned about youth she mused, "They are more civilized than we. . . . They are smarter than we were . . . and they have much more freedom than we had. . . .The only thing I don't like is the way they dress, particularly the girls. They show too much. It's a disgrace." Señora León has never used cosmetics or perfume.

We encountered Belarmino Carpio, eighty-five, as he rode to work astride his donkey and were impressed with the recurrence of the same family name among the elderly—Neptali Carpio, over 100, was another with this same name. Belarmino Carpio had three sons and one daughter, but two of the sons died in infancy (the rate of infant mortality is very high here, as it is in other underdeveloped areas of South America). We watched him light a cigarette made from his own tobacco crop. He uses a stone which he strikes with a piece of metal to produce a spark which in turn ignites a piece of soft, dried cactus stem. His wife is Deifilia Toledo, eighty-six, who bears the family name of another long-lived Vilcabamba family of which José Toledo, age 107, was the patriarch. Belarmino and Deifilia were both born in Vilcabamba and married after a seven-year courtship. They attribute their longevity and vigor to "God and climate." They "almost never eat meat." He says, however, "I smoke and drink a lot."

We traced another elderly Carpio relative, Gabriel Erazo, who lives a short distance outside Vilcabamba but is separated from the village by a mountain trail and rivers which were almost impassable by jeep. Later, on questioning Miguel Carpio about Gabriel Erazo's age, we learned, "He is my cousin and we grew up together. My mother made a big thing out of the fact that we were born the same week (and the same month and same year). In fact, both of us were breast-fed by both mothers, his and mine. When my mother was working, his mother breast-fed both of us, and when his mother was away my mother breast-fed both of us. I heard the story a thousand times from my mother and his mother."

In 1974 I found Gabriel Erazo talkative and delighted to have a big laugh over the urine collection bottle we had given him. Part of our investigation included obtaining twenty-four-hour urine collections from the villagers and he thought this to be a great joke, as did the others. Erazo is small and lean and gets around nimbly with a walking-stick. He always wore a scruffy skullcap, and his tanned and wizened face was animated by shining brown eyes. His face spread into smiles or a hearty laugh at the slightest provocation. He is toothless and has never seen a doctor. He never had any pain and has always been in good health. If he is nearly the same age as Miguel Carpio, as both will attest to, then he appears to have held up much better than his cousin during the four-year interval between our two visits. Since he lives some three hours by horseback over very rough terrain outside of Vilcabamba, the local authorities had arranged for him to stay in the village so as to be available to us during our visit. He was enjoying this vacation greatly and could be found at any time on the town square in conversation with the villagers.

He told us that he makes ropes and that for three *sucre* (about twelve cents) he can make a fifty-foot length of rope, of which he produces two or three per week. He claims to make very good ropes and takes obvious pride in his work. On his farm he grows beans. He arises at 5 A.M. now but used to be up by 4 A.M. His son does the hard work now and he helps. They raise chickens, pigs, and *couhy,* which I found to be guinea pigs, and which are a highly prized delicacy among the villagers. He does not nap during the day and when I tried to determine whether he suffered from the prostatism which so commonly afflicts elder males in our society he admitted that yes, he did have to get up occasionally at night—but because of the fleas!

When asked what was the best time of his life, he replied, "When eggs were cheap and when I went to mass with my parents." He had attended a church school for nearly two years, but when his father died he had to stop and go to work. He had a first child by Juana Deifilia when he was fifteen years old.

Apparently this occurred out of wedlock. He married at age twenty-five to Julia Narvaes, who bore him five children before she died in childbirth some eight years later.

I found Angel Modeste Burneo Valdiezo seated on the front porch of the only post office in Vilcabamba. He was born in Loja and is ninety-one years old. His daughter Gracilia is the postmistress for Vilcabamba, and he now lives with her, taking care of grandchildren and a great-grandson. We were greeted with a cordial embrace by Angel, who is bright eyed, talkative and walks about actively. He now rarely does farm work, and this on a little land some half mile away owned by a son. He was making cigarettes when we found him. He makes approximately 2000 cigarettes daily, of which he smokes about thirty. He has been smoking since the age of eighteen. He claims not to inhale—but as we watched him smoke he exhaled the smoke through his nose. His fingers are deeply stained, and I watched fascinated at their deft and nimble motions rolling the cigarettes. He uses any paper available to wrap the tobacco in. Most of the cigarettes he will sell. I couldn't help notice a flexion contracture of his left little finger which struck me as a strange manifestation of a Dupuytrens contracture. Noticing my puzzlement, he related that at about age twenty-five he was very drunk on one occasion and had tried to shoot himself. He put the pistol to his forehead and pulled the trigger but the gun didn't fire. After a couple more vain attempts he pointed the barrel of the gun at his hand and pulled the trigger. The bullet went through his hand leaving him with the deformity I had noticed. He recounts this episode with much gusto, laughing and gesticulating with enthusiasm. He explained that the local drink is *aguardiente,* distilled from sugar cane and a very potent brew.

When asked the main interest in his life, Angel claims that his first love is living. There were many things that were good, he reminisced. He first fell in love at the age of twenty-five. This woman is still living at age eighty-nine. His second lover has died and the third one, whom he married, has gotten very fat. He claims sex to be very important to a man and added, *"Mujeres magnificas! Matrimonio estupendo!"* He has one son, age seventy, and he himself has been married to his third sweetheart for the past seventy years. He lost his teeth about fifteen years ago, but his vision is still very good.

While others in our group were busy obtaining blood and skin samples I slipped off to hear Dr. Guillermo Vela, nutritionist from Quito and a member of Dr. Salvador's team take a detailed dietary history from ninety-year-old Dolores Mercedes Mendietta Andean. She answered his rapid questions with quick vivacious responses and a smile in her brown lively eyes and wrinkled face. Her gnarled, large-veined hands were farming tools specked with dirt from her last task. Her hair is still very black. She is toothless but wears dentures.

For breakfast she has one glass of milk, bananas fried in lard, sometimes rice, and always bread. After breakfast she washes clothes, runs errands, and goes to church to pray. She never sits down except for her daily half hour in church, and is always busy.

Lunch occurs at about 11 A.M. This consists generally of soup (made from bones, flour, onions, *fideos* [vermicelli], one-half teaspoon of lard, one-half ounce of cheese, and three table-spoons of milk), a glass of milk, potatoes, lettuce ("good for colds"), *lucro,* (a grain) and cocoa with flour and sugar. She used to eat more salt but now takes very little—"It is bad for the kidneys".

After lunch she does not have a siesta as there are too many chores and errands to attend to. Señora Mendietta regards herself as still a shy person. She does not visit friends generally, and if she meets someone she simply exchanges greetings and goes her way.

At 2 P.M. she has a snack consisting of coffee and bread. She admits to a "sweet tooth" and adds one-half to two teaspoons of sugar to each cup of coffee. After this snack she continues her house chores.   She lives in a three-room house and rents one room for fifty *sucre* per month (about $2). There is no water, nor are there toilet facilities. She obtains water from a neighbor and hauls it herself for laundry and other purposes. There is no electricity, and she owns no flashlight. She has no radio. She had learned to read a little as a child but seemed to know almost nothing of politics or current events and was unable to name even one president of Ecuador. She interrupted our queries of current events to ask whether we thought lettuce was good for her.

Supper comes at 4 P.M. This consists of coffee and water with bread. Sometimes she has rice with the bread, "but I always have my bread; it is my life." She prepares rice with water, salt, and lard. Four ounces of rice suffice to make a meal for two. She may also have *fideos,* and onions. If she doesn't eat rice she will have green bananas (*platanos*) fried in a tablespoon of lard.

After this evening meal she goes to church, but if it is bad weather she will do her praying at home. She can recite the litany in Latin. She goes to bed at 9 or 10 P.M. Sometimes she goes right to sleep and other times she prays and thinks until sleep overtakes her.

In summary, her diet includes one-half liter or roughly half a quart, of milk a day, one to two eggs when she can get them—but she has had none for a month. She likes a raw egg in her coffee. She eats cheese approximately three times a week, having one ounce a day when it is available. She loves meat, but she doesn't eat it very often. She had had no meat for fifteen days at the time of this interview; when it is available, one-half pound must last for days. She would eat it daily if she could afford it. Her stomach, she says, doesn't permit her to eat much lard, but she buys four ounces, which will last her for a week. She will have butter once a year under optimal conditions, but she has had none for over a year now. She likes vegetables but gets only tomatoes and lettuce. One head of lettuce will last for one to two days, but she has tomatoes only once a month. She has beans and peppers occasionally but lots of onions. She eats potatoes daily, and one-half pound will last for two meals. Corn she eats occasionally and bread at every meal. Yucca root is a source of starch, but this she has only about once a month because "it bloats her." Rice is eaten three to six times per week, cocoa, legumes, and carrots daily. She likes sweets and buys candies once or twice a month; they will last her for a week each. She cooks for two persons.

She has always been well but has had dentures for the past thirty years. She has been married twice, and her second husband is twenty-five years younger than she. She hasn't lived with him for the past three years, regarding him as a playboy and a ne'er-do-well. She is exceptional in not having any children. Such is the detailed and prosaic account of Dolores Mercedes Mendietta Andean.

In the late afternoon I met Manuel Pardo in the village center returning from work. Manuel claims to be ninety-seven years old. He is slim, toothless, and has an unruly shock of gray hair which stood upright, giving him an alert appearance. He had started for work before the sun came up and worked in the tobacco field of Albertano Roa all that day. He grows some tobacco for himself on another plot of land which he claims is his in addition to this sharecropping for Señor Roa. He is married to his second wife, who is about forty. His youngest child is twelve to fourteen years old.

When asked the most important thing in life, he responded that work was more important than love. The best time of his life was in his youth when everything was cheaper. He feels a person must try everything. He has had very little illness.

I took him to the single "sidewalk cafe" Vilcabamba boasts (one grubby card table) and bought him a beer over which he became quite confidential. He told that his present wife, the woman of forty years, has not been faithful to him. He discovered her with a nephew about two years ago and now he has no more gusto for his work or life. He told how he needed someone for whom he can work in order for his life to be meaningful. When asked what he would do about the situation he said, "I could kill her," but apparently felt that this would not accomplish anything. Although this all happened two years earlier, he is unable to forget it, and his conversation kept returning to this source of his misery. I couldn't help but reflect on the claims I had heard repeatedly that these villagers live such a tranquil, simple life that they have no emotional problems. As is often the case, one finds interpersonal relations are the source of more emotional discomfiture than the stresses of modern living. Manuel Pardo was steeped in the misery of his unfaithful wife.

Another individual whose life in the peaceful valley seemed stressful was Gabriel Sánchez Taday, who claimed to be 102, and whose wife, María Patina Junga Sánchez, was ninety years old. Mr. Sánchez has scanty gray-black hair on his head and a scraggly beard. He is toothless and his high cheekbones and yellow-brown color give him a somewhat oriental appearance. Mr. Sánchez was wrapped up in the injustices that had been perpetrated on him by his landlord. After working for many years, he became very ill some six years ago, at which time the man on whose property he worked threw him off the land. He became very voluble as he recounted this story, gesticulating wildly, and obviously hurt by this experience.

Since being deprived of the land he had cultivated for many years he now works on some community property high on a steep slope on which he raises yucca, corn, and other vegetables. He gets up at sunrise to take care of his few chickens and guinea pigs.

An unmarried daughter who works in a place where coffee is made regularly brings home the lunch with which she is provided, and this supplements the meager diet of Gabriel and his wife. We would have talked longer with Sánchez, but he kept coming back to the injustices perpetrated on him by his patron six years earlier, and we could obtain little other information from him.

I had noticed the intelligent, handsome features of Manuel Ramón in the crowd of old people who were assembled in the school house to greet our arrival on our second visit. When Dr. Elrick and I spoke to him he said he was born in a nearby village nearly 100 years ago. His mother's name was Ennazia Ramón, but he never knew his father. His mother and his only sibling, a sister, had died about forty years ago.

His day begins at 6 A.M. when he breakfasts on coffee with water and yucca. He uses brown sugar in his coffee. He works on a farm high in the hills growing oranges and corn. He has meat once or twice a month, but he has milk daily, as he owns his own cow. He has thirty chickens but sells the eggs and so he eats very few himself. There are three males and two females living in his house whom he identified as his daughter and her son, an adopted son of his own, and his own wife. I became entirely confused in trying to unravel the tangled tale of his own wives and offspring. When asked if he had loves before his first wife, a crafty look came into his eyes and he refused to answer.

In the past everything was cheap and he ate much more meat. The best time he can remember was when he was young and first married. He had once been a cowboy and recounted killing a bear and drinking its blood. This blood ritual we had heard repeated in various form by the superstitious villagers.

I departed from Vilcabamba puzzled as to what was so different in this village from hundreds of other seemingly similar villages in the underdeveloped areas of South America. A subsistence vegetarian diet low in fat content, vigorous physical labor intensified by the mountainous terrain, and the respect of offspring for their parents were hardly unique to Vilcabamba. Because of the apparent family ties linking the elderly in this small enclave of isolated villages, I left with a strong suspicion that genetic factors were of prime importance in explaining the phenomena of successful old age in Vilcabamba.

4

PREVENT OR CURE

There is no short-cut to longevity. To win it is the work of a lifetime, and the promotion of it is a branch of preventive medicine.

Sir James Crichton-Browne (1840–1938), *The Prevention of Senility*

In my introduction I touched briefly on the increasing preoccupation of medicine with treating terminal illness. Curing illness and saving lives has, of course, always been the focus of medicine. Not many years ago the emphasis was almost entirely on the care and relief of suffering. Advances today in our understanding of the biosciences and in technology allow the physician to be concerned mainly with saving lives. This new emphasis has produced brilliant successes with many lives saved. Recent advances in surgery, medical diagnoses, and therapeutics have all contributed to a glamorous and exciting chapter in the long history of medicine. Perhaps it is not accurate to state that this trend represents a new emphasis but rather that new capabilities for actually saving lives have brought this aspect of the physician's activities more into the foreground. I think we would all agree that such an emphasis is appropriate. The first thing we expect and want when we or our loved ones are sick is that the doctor we call will restore us to health as quickly and safely as possible.

But there are times when the will of nature and of the physician are in conflict; and here it is that the physician must perceive when current knowledge and skills are inadequate. Overzealous therapy at this point may be counterproductive to his other obligation to relieve the suffering of his patient. This point is often exceedingly difficult to perceive. Maturity, wisdom, a keen knowledge of his patient, and warm compassion are necessary ingredients in making this decision, which is often a painful one for the physician. These thoughts are well expressed in the statement by F. W. Peabody that, "the secret of the care of the patient is in caring for the patient."

That sustaining life should not always be the sole motivation of the physician was emphasized dramatically by an elderly retired faculty member who called on me shortly after I was appointed chief of medical services at the Massachusetts General Hospital. He wanted me to know that he had lived a long and full life and that, should he be stricken and brought into my hospital, he didn't want to be stuck with needles nor have his bodily orifices stuffed with tubes. He wanted to be allowed to die in comfort and in dignity. If any of my young doctors attempted to put needles into him, he warned that he would take the needles and stick them into the doctors! The patient today is often denied a dignified death because of the zeal to preserve life. There is a time when every effort is justified and should be made, but also there is a time when such efforts are inappropriate and no longer in the patient's interest.

The responsibility of the physician is primarily to his patient. This relationship is time honored and respected. One aspect of this bond is the confidentiality of communication between patient and physician which has attained legal status. But increasingly today one sees the clash between the obligation of the physician to his patient as an individual and societal interests. Such conflicts arise from the almost limitless resources which medical care may consume in the treatment of desperately ill patients. With technology that can keep the heart beating and sustain respiration almost indefinitely in many instances, the temptation is to battle to the end in the perceived interests of trying to save the patient's life. Blood banks may be exhausted, expensive antibiotics, hormones, and other medications consumed, repeated surgical procedures performed, organs transplanted, hospital beds and personnel taxed to the limit before the death of the patient stops the effort. Although near-miracles are often performed by such efforts, there are times when the outcome is doomed to failure nearly from the start. This is particularly true in the elderly or debilitated who lack the reserve to sustain and support themselves through a failure of some bodily system.

Recently I attended a conference of surgeons and internists to consider what measures might be taken to improve the dismal outcome of patients who came to the hospital as emergencies having already ruptured an abdominal aortic aneurysm. The aorta is the major artery carrying blood from the heart with branches to head, trunk, and extremities. It is prone to atherosclerosis. Atherosclerosis causes weakness of the aortic wall, which, fortunately, only in rare instances will progress to ballooning and finally rupture or tear. Loss of blood into surrounding tissues may occur gradually or quickly, but the patient generally is in shock from blood loss by the time he arrives at the hospital or shortly thereafter. It is customary in most centers to resort to emergency surgery. Surgery involves cross-clamping the aorta above the site of rupture, excising the affected portion of aorta, and reestablishing continuity with a graft of synthetic plastic. When the diagnosis of impending rupture can be made early, this procedure is of proven prophylactic value, but when rupture has occurred prior to surgery the patient is in a very precarious situation, and the likelihood that he will be able to survive surgery and the postoperative period is very limited. In fact, two series of surgically treated patients were discussed. The first included forty patients, of whom only one survived to leave the hospital. The hospital costs for these forty patients totaled over a million dollars. Of the next twenty-three patients, nineteen died and four survived; the cost for each survival was $93,000. The reason that I cite the costs is not to make a judgment regarding the price of a human life but to emphasize the enormous costs and use of rare resources which can be consumed in an effort to save a life in just one of the many overwhelming medical disasters which can occur.

If one notes further that in the particular sample I have cited the average age of the patients was seventy, one can realize the futility of the curative approach in dealing with such an over-whelming catastrophe, regardless of the skills and resources that are applied. With age there is an increase in the number of pathologic changes which affect several systems or organs in the body. Thus a patient with atherosclerosis of such a severe degree to lead to local rupture of the abdominal aorta is likely to have extensive vascular disease affecting the coronary arteries of his heart and the carotid and cerebral vessels which supply his brain; in addition, he may also have limitation of his pulmonary function, chronic liver or kidney disease, and so forth. The condition which has produced manifest disease at one site is likely to have increased the likelihood that a similar disease will strike elsewhere. This is certainly true of diseases of the blood vessels but may also be true in the case of inflammatory processes or cancer. Most people who die late in life from one of these causes also exhibit several other pathological processes which would probably have killed them very soon had they survived the actual cause of their death. Alex Comfort has pointed out that the characteristic pathological feature of aging is an increase in the number of pathological changes present. This makes the likelihood of success very small if we expend all our efforts and resources in trying to cure each pathologic process as its clinical manifestations surface—which they will, and with increasing frequency.

Medicine needs to save lives and relieve suffering where

possible, but physicians must develop clearer criteria for prognosis and treat dying patients on the basis of probable benefit from treatment rather than throw every therapeutic measure available into the breech regardless of the likelihood of a successful outcome. Today we have the capabilities to save some lives which only a few years ago would have been hopelessly lost. Now medical teams in major centers are tackling the problems of even sicker patients. Worthwhile as such progress may be, the effort and resources expended increase exponentially as the margin of benefit to the individual and to society diminishes.

There is no escape from the inevitable logic of this dilemma—as the effort increases the benefit diminishes. Thus, it seems to be timely to reappraise the directions we. are taking, examine our present posture, and decide whether the current course is the most advantageous to all or whether some alternative approach should command the attention and energies of more of the medical profession. I believe the latter to be the case. As I see the ravages of disease attain irreversible stages, the futility of the curative approach even for the afflicted individual becomes often painfully apparent. Coronary bypass surgery, for example, cannot solve the national health problem posed by heart attacks which have reached epidemic proportions in our society today and strike down increasing numbers of males at early ages. We must learn the causes of this and other killers and prevent their occurrence. Only in prevention is there hope of adding significant vigorous years to our lives.

Many physicians today are skeptical about substantially benefiting the national health or even the individual's health significantly through the practice of preventive medicine. This skepticism has several causes. It is often difficult to detect early stages of disease and for many of the chronic disease killers there is all too little that we know that can be done to halt their progression. Too many crusades to make the public aware of early clues to the presence of disease may create a state of national hypochondriasis. Even the annual checkup has its detractors. The advice of the physician "to lose a little weight", "stop smoking", "get some regular exercise", "eat regular nutritious meals", "stop worrying so much", "cut down on the alcohol", and "get more rest" rarely affects life-long habits of eating, drinking, smoking, physical indolence, and worry until the disease process is so apparent that heeding the oft-repeated admonitions can no longer help. Furthermore, the roots of many of our illnesses lie so deep in the social and economic structure of our country that most doctors find them beyond the range of their medical competence. The patient with alcoholic cirrhosis can be kept from his alcohol, offered a nutritious diet, and treated for an excess of body fluids in the hospital. But on discharge he is likely to return to his former life—including the alcohol and irregular meals which are gradually destroying his liver and his life. It is true that more and more doctors work together with social workers and agencies, who make great efforts to improve the social environment of the patient after he leaves the hospital. Valiant and worthwhile as such efforts are, they are unlikely to reduce the net poverty, malnutrition, and unhappiness in the community, and thus they fail to affect the breeding sources of further illness.

The doctor today stands at the end of the line, coping as best as he can with all his skill and training with the diseased or wrecked lives that come to him. The physician rightly perceives that his training has given him very little advantage over any other educated citizen in correcting society's ills. He is soon so engrossed and overworked with his efforts in curative medicine that he has little energy left (and often too little interest) to devote himself to preventive or prophylactic measures, whether they be medical, social, or economic. Finally, he is well remunerated by society for sticking to what he has been trained so well to do—provide curative medicine to the sick.

The rewards in a fee-for-service system such as ours are all for practicing curative medicine, and no body of physicians in the long history of medicine is more knowledgeable and skillful in the curative arts than our physicians of today. But the nature of the chronic illnesses which are now the major killers and responsible also for most of the debility and senility of our aged are not likely to yield to curative medicine—they have caused too much irreversible damage often by the time they are discovered. We need a whole new approach to prevention of illness.

First, a great deal more research is needed on the aging process itself; what happens to cells, molecules, tissue, and organs with time must be understood before we can know what the optimal conditions of life are which would minimize the adverse effects of time on the living organism. The biology of aging is discussed in detail elsewhere, but clearly our knowledge of the subject is at an early stage and only beginning to attract the interest of scientists and the financial support that can lead to rapid progress.

Second, a great deal more research is needed into the causes of the chronic illnesses which exact their toll chiefly among the elderly. Effective programs of prevention must be based upon a clear understanding of cause. Arteriosclerosis, cancer, and hypertension are the major malefactors. Arteriosclerosis, which is the proximate cause of both heart attacks and strokes, is currently receiving increasing attention, as is cancer research.

Support for research in these areas has been forthcoming primarily through our National Institutes of Health. This support should in time provide the answers that are needed. However, much of the understanding that is required is at a very fundamental level, and nature reveals her basic secrets slowly, even to the prepared mind which asks the right questions.

There has been a tendency for the public to become impatient with the pace of scientific progress related to our understanding of diseases. This reveals itself through the political process which controls government expenditures for research. Recently research budgets have been slashed and support for the training of young scientists sharply curtailed by the Administration in Washington. Availability of research support has been tied to huge, cumbersome bureaucratic schemes imposed on the scientific community in hopes of ordering a more rapid pace of research accomplishments. Organized, targeted research programs may be effective in hastening practical results where the basic scientific understanding already exists; the development of the atomic bomb during the Second World War is a case in point. But, where the basic principles still remain to be discovered, contractual targeted research programs are likely to be expensive and counterproductive. Support and freedom to pursue his ideas provide the optimal environment for the creative scientist. It is the difficulty of the problems, not the lack of industry or motivation, which retards the pace of understanding. The clamor for immediate practical results from the large research projects supported by our National Cancer Institute and National Heart and Lung Institute is likely to divert effort and resources from the search for basic knowledge without which crash programs are doomed to failure. The unregimented scientist will be the most creative one, and there remains a great need for much creative science in these important areas of health research.

Third, understanding of how to improve health must be more effectively translated into positive public action. This has been a particularly frustrating matter to all physicians and health workers. How does one influence people to change their behavior so as to live according to what will favor preservation of their good health? This question is a pressing one not only in introducing positive new factors which will improve health but for an age in which we haven't even learned how to motivate people not to adopt measures which are patently self-destructive—witness the recent rise in drug addiction.

At a Senate hearing on the need for federal support for medical research, a very distinguished medical scientist recently testified. In response to a direct question from a senator regarding what practical applications had come from the important discoveries he had made, the scientist responded, "We [the medical research community] have proven that cigarette smoking is injurious to health. When you [senators] have abolished cigarette smoking then I'll be happy to tell you what next to work on. In the meantime allow me to continue my basic research and don't worry whether it will produce immediate practical benefits." Undoubtedly such remarks sound arrogant in the extreme; but they do emphasize the dilemma we face. The public expects a pill or an inoculation to be the practical outcome of the health-related research. But if the promotion of health requires major changes in living habits then the public acceptance and response is at best sluggish. Since cigarette smoking has been proven to be a cause of lung cancer and a factor in heart disease and in chronic lung disease, there has been a striking reduction in smoking among physicians, but the sale of cigarettes in our country has not decreased. Does one have to educate all the public to the level of physicians in order to get the public to perceive the need to quit smoking cigarettes? Clearly there will have to be some less expensive means of persuasion—but what is it? Research on this urgent matter of influencing behavior in support of the individual's best interests is needed. It is to be hoped that this can be done through means which are based on enlightened self-interest rather than upon compulsion.

Fourth, we must have a health care system based on prepayment rather than fee-for-service. By prepayment I am referring to a system of health insurance in which the subscriber pays an annual premium to cover a broad spectrum of services. The physicians who provide these services are not reimbursed according to the services rendered. They may be paid reasonable salaries, which will remove any personal conflict of interest in performing unnecessary, expensive procedures or services. Alternatively, they may be salaried with bonuses paid based on the savings in cost to the program which accrue from the reduced utilization of expensive medical facilities. For example, many diagnostic studies can be performed on an ambulatory basis, avoiding the large expense that hospitalization entails. Most medical insurance plans, however, will only pay for procedures performed during hospitalization. The effect of this reimbursement system is often to drive patients into the hospital for procedures which could be performed much less expensively in the office.

The most effective means of reducing costs is to keep the subscribers to the plan healthy. Thus the reward to the physician is changed from providing costly services to the patient only after illness has struck to providing prevention which will avoid costly services. Such health insurance may be provided by a private insurer, such as the Kaiser Health Plan, or in more comprehensive coverage by a national health service, such as that of Great Britain. In the first instance it is based on a voluntary subscription with premiums paid directly to the insurer; in the latter, it is compulsory and supported by taxation.

There is adequate documentation that a prepaid health care system can create a fiscal motivation for the physician to keep his patient healthy and thus avoid hospitalization. The present fee-for-service system retains the emphasis of the physician's activities on the curative aspects of illness. Such an approach can't meet with notable successes in the case of just those diseases that are most inimicable to a long healthy life, as stressed earlier.

With all the public discussion regarding the chaos existing in our health care delivery system and the best solution to the rising costs of medical care, its lack of availability to many, and its maldistribution, the issue of fee-for-service looms as central. Organized medicine has stalwartly fought for preservation of a fee-for-service system. It has supported various health insurance schemes so long as these have preserved the principle of fee-for-service. In doing this organized medicine has recognized a major fiscal incentive in the practice of medicine. But as long as this incentive is by fee-for-service it cannot provide a force to alter the present emphasis on curative practice. In fact, it is a mode of remuneration ideally suited to preserve the practice of medicine in its present mold.

Today it is fashionable to blame the medical schools for the present unsatisfactory state of medical care in our country. The medical schools are blamed for teaching the wrong subjects, too much science, too little practical work, training too many specialists, academicians, and investigators and not enough doctors willing to go out into general medical practice to bring to the public the advantages modern medicine has to offer. I believe such accusations are ill directed. How medicine is practiced is much more influenced by the practicalities of the marketplace than by the curriculum in the medical schools. I had the opportunity to talk to medical educators and public health officials in Great Britain and Sweden, where national health services provide at least ready access for all citizens to the health care system, and the disaffection so prevalent in the United States does not exist in those countries. I asked these officials how much they had to change their medical educational system in order to provide the physicians needed by their national health services. They were quite surprised by my question, as there had been no changes made; their medical education has remained much more traditional than ours. It is only very recently—years after their national health services were going concerns—that innovations in education which increase emphasis on the teaching of ambulatory medicine have been introduced.

A prepayment health service, with a fiscal incentive for physicians and allied health workers to keep the public healthy and out of the expensive hospitals, would, I believe, do much to direct attention of the medical profession toward better methods of preventive medicine. The Chinese recognized this principle long ago in a traditional system which paid the physician for keeping them healthy and ceased payment when illness occurred; illness was regarded as a failure on the part of the physician. The view may have been extreme, but the emphasis I believe to be correct.

In summary, I quote Huang Ti (the Yellow Emperor—2697–2597 B.C.): "Hence the sages did not treat those who were already ill; they instructed those who were not yet ill. . . . To administer medicines to diseases which have already developed and to suppress revolts which have already developed is comparable to the behavior of those persons who begin to dig a well after they have become thirsty, and of those who begin to cast weapons after they have already engaged in battle."

NUTRITION

They are as sick that surfeit with too much as they starve
with nothing.

William Shakespeare (1564–1616),
The Merchant of Venice, I, ii, 6

Since we are composed of what we eat and drink, it is not surprising that diet holds a primary position in discussions of health and longevity. Certainly malnutrition, together with infections, has been the major cause of a reduced life span throughout man's existence. The two scourges, malnutrition and infections, have been mutually reinforcing. The study of nutrition and improvements in the availability of foods, as well as public health and sanitary measures, have made the most significant contributions to the extension of the mean life span in industrially advanced societies. Today, with our stores filled with food products, we are tending to the opposite extreme: we impair health and reduce longevity by overeating. Eighty percent of Americans are overweight. It has been aptly stated that many of us dig our graves with a fork.

DIETARY REQUIREMENTS

The Food and Nutrition Board of the U.S. Academy of Sciences–National Research Council in 1968 recommended 2400 calories with 65 grams of protein for males over fifty-five, and 1700 calories with 55 grams of protein for females aged fifty-five and above. The actual daily food intake recorded in 1965 by the Agricultural Research Service of the U.S. Department of Agriculture was found to be:

	Age	Calories	Protein	Fat	Carbohydrate
Male	55–64	2422	98 grams	121 grams	227 grams
	64–74	2058	83	101	203
	75+	1870	73	90	191
Female	55–64	1619	67 grams	80 grams	158 grams
	65–74	1473	60	70	151
	75+	1459	59	68	154

Thus the actual ingested calories are close to the recommended values for the first decade after age fifty-five. However, the higher protein intake reflects the high contribution of meats to our diets.

In contrast to these figures for the elderly in the United States, Dr. Maqsood Ali found in a nutritional survey of the diets of fifty-five male adults in Hunza an average daily caloric intake of 1923 calories, with 50 grams of protein, 35 grams of fat, and 354 grams of carbohydrate. Furthermore, meat and dairy products constituted only one percent of the total. The absence of pasture land makes animal husbandry nearly impossible. The few cattle are killed for food during the winter and on festive occasions.

Fats of animal origin are indeed scarce, not by preference, we noted, as we watched with amazement while a pound or so of butter, which we had graciously declined, quickly disappeared, swallowed in large chunks by our guide and driver. It obviously was regarded as a rare delicacy.

Oil obtained from the seeds of apricots is generally used for all culinary purposes in Hunza. We watched with fascination as ninety-five-year-old Niay Bibi and her seventy-five-year-old daughter Dault Bibi of Hyderabad village demonstrated for us the method by which the oil is obtained. First the seeds are ground to a fine meal in a communal mortar (a nine- to ten-inch round hole worn in a large rock in the middle of a path) with a large stone pestle. The meal is then kneaded to a paste in a shallow, heavy earthen dish which has been heated over an open fire. Water is added to the paste to maintain a proper consistency. The paste is vigorously kneaded by both bare hands (nothing mentioned in the directions about cleanliness!)—and suddenly large amounts of fragrant oil ooze forth from the mess. Continued kneading and squeezing of the pulp gives a good yield of aromatic, almond-scented oil. The mash remaining is also eaten as a special dish. A word of warning is necessary to any who may wish to try extracting oil from apricot kernels themselves. The kernels of apricots in Hunza are free of the very poisonous cyanide which is a natural constituent of apricot and peach kernels in this country. Highly lethal amounts of cyanide may be encountered in attempts to extract oils from the kernels of American apricots or peaches.

Dr. Guillermo Vela, a nutritionist of Quito, Ecuador, also found a strikingly low caloric consumption among the elderly of Vilcabamba. The average daily diet yielded 1200 calories, with a maximal figure of 1360 calories. The daily protein intake is 35 to 38 grams, with fat comprising only 12 to 19 grams; 200 to 360 grams of carbohydrate complete the diet. Protein and fat again are largely of vegetable origin, with only some 12 grams of protein daily from animal sources. Little or no undernutrition is seen in these communities. Needless to say, one sees no obesity among the elderly in either Vilcabamba or Hunza, whereas both health and aesthetics are constantly violated in our society by caloric excess.

The weight of current medical opinion would concur that a diet such as that described for Hunza and Vilcabamba would delay development of atherosclerosis. Confidence in the importance to health and longevity of a low animal fat, low cholesterol, and low caloric diet is somewhat shaken, however, by eating habits in the Caucasus. Dr. Deli Dzhorbenzdze and Professor G. Z. Pitzkhelauri have studied the dietary habits of 9304 persons over the age of eighty, including 625 centenarians. The old people consume 1700 to 1900 calories daily, which is less than the 2000 calories the Central Institute of Nutrition of Russia recommends for old people. No special diet is eaten by the elderly. Sixty percent eat a mixed diet with milk, vegetables, meats, and fruit. Seventy percent of the calories are of vegetable origin and the remainder from meat and dairy products. Aside from the increased vegetable intake and diminished meat which the senile or sick choose, there is no evidence of dietary selection in relation to health. Seventy to ninety grams of protein are included in the diets. Milk is a main source of protein, with sour milk and cheese widely used in all meals and at all seasons. Georgian cheeses are low in fat content; thus the daily fat intake is only 40 to 60 grams. In eastern Georgia butter is eaten, but in the west vegetable oils rather than butter are used. About thirty percent of dietary fat is of vegetable origin; the remainder is animal fat.

Bread provides the major source of carbohydrates. In central Georgia marvelous long flat pointed loaves resembling Saracen slippers turned up at both ends, two feet or so in length, are baked in an outside oven and stacked, while still crisp and warm, on the table. In the west, a flat, unraised, soft white loaf is eaten. Also in the west, *mamaligia,* a heavy, boiled, white, unflavored corn meal mush patty, is eaten with the fingers and dipped into a variety of spicy sauces or sharp red pepper. Hot spices are favored by the elderly, who claim that appetite and digestion benefit therefrom.

Breakfast generally consists of cheese, bread, and tea; much honey is eaten. The usual beverage is sour milk with cold water added. Tea is also drunk. Every household has its vineyard and makes its own wine, which is quite dry and drunk fresh. The old people consume two to three glasses daily with their meals, and far greater quantities at feasts or festivals.

These festivities hardly seemed consistent with the habits of moderation which we were told the old people exercised. However, though the centenarians generally participated in all aspects of the banquet, one noted that often they would forego the vodka and that their wineglasses were smaller than ours. I never did ascertain whether their habits had always been so moderate or whether the moderation was only acquired in old age. At age fifty, sixty, or seventy, were they drinking and eating like the others at the table? From what we saw I believe so, but of course such feasts were not a daily event, nor was food always so plentiful. We were often told by the old people that "things are much better now." When asked to explain this statement one Armenian replied, "In Turkey and when we first came here, we had only beans and some vegetables to eat, but now we have meat and wine every day." It is well documented in animal experiments that a low-calorie diet during early life will extend the total life span. Thus dietary habits during early life may be more pertinent to longevity than moderation exercised in old age.

When we drove to the village of Chloy we found Tandel Dschopia dressed in full Abkhasian native costume waiting for us under the trees. He looked no more than seventy-five years old—a big, handsome, lean man with a vigorous and authoritative bearing. He proved to be 102 or 103. After a long interview followed by a very vigorous demonstration of his dancing, he apologized that he would not join us at the sumptuous feast which the collective farm had prepared in our honor. When the others present laughed at this announcement by Tandel the following explanation was elicited. Apparently our visit had been expected two days earlier. After waiting from 10 A.M. to 8 P.M., however, the villagers, including Tandel, decided to go ahead with the festivities which they had prepared. They drank that night until midnight. After a few short hours of rest the drinking resumed and continued all day. It was understandable that Tandel was reluctant to join the merriment this day, and I marveled even more at the display of native dances which he performed with such vigor in the midday heat.

In the countryside only the adult males sit at table during such festivities. The women and children wait on table, and, though they keep an interested eye on the proceedings, they do not participate. Only where there were centenarians among the women of the household did they join us at table. Since a household includes not one family but the families of sons, daughters, grandchildren, and other close relatives who may have their houses built next to one another, there may be three to five houses comprising the household group.

In Vilcabamba and Hunza the old people were generally quite slim, but in Georgia we saw an occasional obese centenarian, a phenomenon I would not have thought possible. On a farm near Gulripshi we visited Quada Jonashia, who is a 110-year-old Armenian. He told us, "If one is healthy, it is obligatory to drink one liter of wine daily, and on holidays and weddings seventeen to twenty tumblers are common." He eats everything and is definitely obese now, but both he and his grandson claim he was much fatter a few years earlier. Sonchka Kvetzenia of Atara is 107 and very fat. When I tried to inquire diplomatically how long she had been overweight, she laughed and said, "I became fat when I stopped having children. For sixty years I have been fat as a barrel and all my children are like me. My mother was fatter, stronger, and warmer than I!" We learned that her mother had died only recently and had been the oldest person in that region at the time of her death. These obese people, of course, are the exceptions, but nevertheless striking to this physician, who was taught and has taught that obesity is an unmitigated health disaster. However, recent epidemiologic studies in this country indicate that moderate obesity is not a marked risk factor; at least it is not as dangerous as hypertension, elevated serum cholesterol, or the smoking of twenty or more cigarettes daily. It is probably largely through the hypertension, elevated blood fats, or diabetes so often associated with obesity that obesity becomes a risk factor for heart attacks.

If we set aside these unusual instances of obesity and longevity, the general dietary pattern in the three areas visited conforms with current medical thinking. A sufficient number of calories should be provided, with ample vitamins, minerals, essential amino acids, and fatty acids to meet all the body's needs. Obviously toxic substances must be avoided, such as pesticides on fruits or vegetables, heavy metals such as in mercury contamination of certain seafoods, and bacterial contaminants. The dietary contribution to failure of optimal health in affluent societies may be due to a deficient intake of some essential dietary ingredient, an excess of imbalance of diet, or the unwitting ingestion of toxins with the diet. Clearly all three possibilities may interfere with optimal health, and each has constituted focal positions from which dietary fads have been launched repeatedly over the centuries.

DIET AND DISEASE

It is well recognized that diet has a profound effect on patterns of disease. This fact is immediately apparent if one considers the high incidence of death and disease among the young due to infection in undernourished populations and, conversely, the high frequency in older individuals of heart disease and cancer in well-fed affluent societies. The relation of diet to cardiovascular disease, the leading killer in our country, has been the subject of many studies. The underlying pathologic changes in the blood vessels when atherosclerosis affects the cerebral, cardiac, or peripheral circulations are virtually identical. Arteriosclerosis is a chronic disease of blood vessels in which thickening and hardening of arterial walls interferes with the circulation of the blood. Atherosclerosis is a form of arteriosclerosis affecting primarily the large arteries but also the arteries of heart and brain. It is characterized by deposits or degenerative accumulations of pulpy, acellular lipid and calcium-containing materials in arterial walls, which thicken the arterial wall so as to narrow and gradually obstruct the cavity of the vessel. The Framingham Study has identified several factors which seem to contribute to the occurrence of atherosclerotic disease. The factors are high blood pressure, elevated serum cholesterol, intolerance to glucose, cigarette smoking, and electrocardiographic evidence of hypertrophy (enlargement) of the left ventricle of the heart. The electrocardiographic changes are undoubtedly the result of hypertension and atherosclerosis rather than their cause.

Salt and Blood Pressure

The consideration of dietary factors in relationship to hypertension (high blood pressure) has been dominated by a possible role for sodium chloride (common table salt). A convincing argument can be derived from epidemiologic and experimental studies to implicate excessive salt intake as an important causative factor in hypertension. Recently a six-year study of tribal societies in the Solomon Islands has concluded that Solomon Islanders rarely have high blood pressure, but that highest pressures occur in the tribe with the highest salt intake. In anephric patients (patients without kidney function who are being kept alive by dialysis) the blood pressure has been found to be sensitive to the sodium balance, rising with an increase in the content of salt in the body and decreasing upon removal of salt by dialysis. However, the correlations are rough, and the suspicion exists that other pathologic factors are necessary to sensitize blood vessels to the effects of sodium, sodium excess being generally a necessary but insufficient cause of hypertension.

L. K. Dahl has long been a proponent of the causal role of sodium in human vascular hypertension. He bases his belief on an undeniable clinical observation that adherence to a very low dietary sodium intake will reduce the blood pressure of most hypertensive patients. In its extreme form such a diet may be restricted to boiled rice and fruits, as advocated by Klempner, but it is the very low sodium intake rather than other peculiarities of the composition of the diet that is the important factor in reducing blood pressure. The introduction of diuretic agents, which enhance the excretion of salt by the kidneys and lower blood pressure, is predicated on the same basis—namely, that a modest reduction in the body content of sodium favors a lower blood pressure. Of course a drastic loss of body sodium, as may occur with severe diarrhea—e.g., with cholera—or with excessive sweating, can so compromise the blood volume that circulation cannot be sustained; blood pressure falls and vascular collapse, shock and death may ensue.

The demonstration that our customary high salt diet is causally related to the high incidence of hypertension has not been so generally accepted. A very high salt intake will cause an elevation of blood pressure in relatively few normal persons. But Dahl points out that such experiments are of short duration compared with our lifetime dietary habits of adding salt to our foods. He points out that man had developed for ages before salt became a common dietary constituent. Natural foods are low in sodium. Persons who are primarily vegetarians might average 2 to 10 milliequivalents of sodium (0.1 to 0.6 grams as sodium chloride) per day; whereas those who are primarily meat-eaters would average more, since meat contains the sodium in the body fluids of the prey. However, only if the meat intake provided as much as 4000 calories per day would the sodium intake approximate the

10 grams of salt so commonly exceeded in our foods today. The body can deal so economically with sodium and conserve its content of sodium so efficiently that the daily requirements for an adult are as low as 5 milliequivalents (0.25 grams of table salt, about one-sixteenth of a level teaspoonful!). The average American diet by contrast contains about 10 grams of salt daily with a large variation from day to day—and even more, as the total varies from individual to individual from perhaps 4 to 24 grams. Even those who do not use a salt shaker at the table acquire a considerable intake from processed foods or salt added during cooking.

Although there is great individual variability in the blood pressure response to a high salt intake, epidemiologic studies—that is, the study of populations in relation to incidence of disease—reveal a relationship between the average quantity of sodium ingested by a population and the incidence of hypertension. The higher the salt intake the higher the proportion of hypertensive individuals in the population. The Solomon Islanders, Eskimos, and certain primitive tribes have a much lower sodium content in their diets than ours and less hypertension. In Japan, especially in the north, salt intake is very high, even by our standards, and hypertension and strokes are very common.

Dahl emphasizes that hypertension has several causal ingredients. He has found that, by subjecting rats to a high sodium diet, some rats will become hypertensive and others seem not to develop hypertension. By selectively inbreeding rats which respond to a high salt intake by developing hypertension he has succeeded in developing a strain which is highly sensitive to salt intake. Similarly, a salt-resistant nonhypertensive strain was produced by inbreeding the nonresponsive rats. With these two strains of rats the interaction of genetic and environmental factors in the occurrence of hypertension is clearly manifested. Neither group develops hypertension when the environmental factor, sodium, is lacking. When the diet provides a high salt intake the hypertension appears in those who had the genetic susceptibility of sensitivity to salt. Dahl believes that a similar combination of genetic and environmental factors may be involved in most human subjects with arterial hypertension. This would account for the higher incidence of hypertension among members of cultures that customarily ingest large amounts of salt. It would explain also why only an occasional normal person develops hypertension experimentally on a high salt intake.

How a high salt intake contributes to elevation of the arterial blood pressure in the susceptible individual is not clear. Whether it is the small overexpansion of the circulating blood volume that is the major effect or whether the excess sodium increases the resistance of blood vessels through some more direct effect on the caliber of the small arteries remains uncertain. What seems certain, however, is that for the major degenerative diseases—hypertension, atherosclerosis, senile dementia, and cancer—multiple etiologic (causal) factors are involved. The continued search for a single causal factor in these conditions is unlikely to succeed. Generally a concurrence of genetic and environmental factors in the same individual will be required. However, there is always a danger that, when several different factors are involved in the etiology, the glib rationalist can easily explain any situation that may arise and other important factors may be overlooked.

Diet and Heart Attacks

Investigations have focused on the blood lipids (fats), especially cholesterol, in atherosclerosis. That an association between cholesterol and atherosclerosis exists is undeniable; whether it is a causal relationship still is based largely on guilt by association. Nevertheless, the associations are so manifold as to raise a high probability of a causal link between the two: (1) Persons with high blood cholesterol levels have been found in epidemiologic studies to develop coronary heart disease with greater frequency than those with lower levels; (2) The elevation of serum cholesterol (hypercholesterolemia) precedes the development of coronary heart disease, and the risk of the latter is proportional to the degree of elevation of the blood cholesterol; (3) Diseases associated with hypercholesterolemia are associated with premature atherosclerosis, as in Type II hyperlipidemia (a hereditary condition in which blood lipids are markedly elevated), a genetically determined hyperlipidemia; (4) Populations with high average blood cholesterol concentrations have a higher occurrence of coronary deaths than those with low cholesterol levels; (5) The large quantities of cholesterol within the atheromatous lesions have long been recognized and the movement of cholesterol from the blood into such lesions has been demonstrated (atheromatous lesions are the plaques of acellular lipid- and calcium-containing material deposited in the walls of arteries); (6) Atherosclerosis can be produced in certain animals by the dietary induction of high blood cholesterol levels, and the atheromatous deposits can be made to regress by dietary manipulations which lower the cholesterol level (for example, Rhesus monkeys subjected to high-fat, high-cholesterol diets showed significant coronary atheromatosis at the end of seventeen months; when subsequently placed on a cholesterol-free diet for forty months, regression of the coronary atheromatosis was demonstrated with an average increase in cross-sectional area (the lumen) of the coronary arteries of more than eighty percent—though it should be stated that some authorities have questioned whether the lesions produced in monkeys are really identical with the atherosclerosis found in man); (7) In man, prospective studies have shown that diets restricted in saturated fats and cholesterol reduced the recurrence of heart attacks in male survivors of initial myocardial infarcts; the relapse rate correlated with the serum cholesterol level maintained during the trial—the higher the cholesterol, the higher the relapse rate; (8) Primary protection against the initial development of coronary heart disease by diets which lower blood cholesterol has also been demonstrated. Such is the nature and abundance of the data linking cholesterol to atherosclerosis.

The role of the diet in controlling heart attacks seems now well established. The evidence comes from two types of studies: studies on the prevention of initial heart attacks (primary prevention) and studies aimed at preventing recurrences of heart attacks (secondary prevention). Experiments of the second type are easier to perform, since subjects who have experienced one heart attack are more likely to volunteer to a marked change in their diets and adhere to the program than individuals who have experienced no cardiac problems. Since the likelihood of a recurrent heart attack is much greater than an initial attack in the population at large, a smaller group of subjects is required to establish a statistically significant result. Nevertheless, conclusions from these two kinds of studies need not necessarily be interchangeable. Once involvement of coronary arteries by the atheromatous process is sufficiently extensive to produce a heart attack the process may be too far advanced to be halted or reversed by dietary or other means. Nonetheless, results have shown that a diet which effectively lowers the serum cholesterol is beneficial in both primary and secondary prevention of heart attacks. Several dietary experiments may be cited.

A five-year study in Norway by Paul Leren was a preventative trial among 412 male survivors of heart attacks in the age range from thirty to sixty-seven years which began in 1958. The treatment group received a diet low in saturated fats and cholesterol with increased amounts of polyunsaturated fats. This was accomplished by almost complete elimination of fat of meat and milk origin. Only one egg per week was permitted and liberal quantities of soybean oil—an unsaturated oil—were recommended. Adherence to the diet was checked by means of a questionnaire, and the control group was also interrogated about its eating habits.

The serum cholesterol levels in this group of males who had experienced a heart attack were unusually high, averaging nearly 300 mgs per 100 ml (250 mgs per 100 ml of serum is generally regarded as the upper limit of normal). The diet designed to reduce the serum cholesterol was successful, as indicated by a sustained drop in serum cholesterol levels in the treatment group. This decrease averaged about 40 mgs per 100 ml for the duration of the study.

The effectiveness of the dietary intervention was assessed by three criteria: occurrence of new heart attacks, development of angina pectoris (the squeezing chest pain characteristic of inadequate blood supply to the muscle of the heart), and sudden deaths. The number of patients with coronary relapses by these three criteria was significantly lower in the diet group with fewer recurrent heart attacks and acquired angina pectoris. A closer examination of the figures reveals that the preventive effect of the diet was highly significant in the age group below sixty years but not in the older subjects. The most striking beneficial effect was seen in those who had recovered from their previous heart attack with no obvious signs or symptoms of heart disease. Furthermore, the relapse rates were definitely correlated with the level of serum cholesterol maintained during the study; the higher the cholesterol, the higher the relapse rate.

Another major test of the low cholesterol, increased polyunsaturated fat diet was conducted by S. Dayton and associates on 846 middle-aged and elderly men living in the domiciliary unit of the Los Angeles Veterans Adminstration Center. Of these, one-half received the conventional diet as control and the other half the experimental diet low in saturated fats and cholesterol. Adherence over the entire period was monitored in terms of dining-room attendance records.

Volunteers were accepted into the study regardless of possible preexisting atherosclerotic complications. A subject was considered a participant from the day he was assigned to diet until termination of the trial or until death, regardless of possible absence from the Center or noncooperation during the interval. Adherence over the entire period of the trial accordingly amounted to fifty-six percent of total possible meals for the control subjects and forty-seven percent for the experimental group. The study commenced in 1959 and included a period of eight years of exposure to the diets. Serum cholesterols on the average were the same for the two groups but fell by 12.7 percent in the experimental dietary group. The combined incidence of myocardial infarction, sudden death, and stroke was significantly lower in the experimental group than in the control group. The incidence of fatal atherosclerotic events was also lower in the experimental group than in the control group, but total mortality rates were similar for the two groups. This latter fact is not surprising, since the study included a sizable group of elderly subjects (fifty percent were over 65.5 years old). The authors concluded that this trial leads to the qualified conclusion that lowering of serum cholesterol levels by the dietary means employed can lower the incidence of atherosclerotic complications in men aged fifty-four to sixty-five, but not necessarily at more advanced ages. The possibility that an increased incidence of cancers in the experimental group was caused by the increased intake of polyunsaturated fatty acids seems adequately negated by subsequent studies.

A third study of secondary prevention was reported in 1967 by M. L. Bierenbaum and associates. Their study was a five-year study in two groups of fifty men aged thirty to fifty with coronary artery disease who were given one of two different low-fat diets. A matched control group of 100 men with coronary artery disease was recruited. The results showed a statistically significant decrease in fatal myocardial infarctions in men less than forty-five years of age who were on the experimental low-fat diets as compared with the control group.

Another major study, however, failed to show a beneficial effect of a serum cholesterol lowering diet in the prevention of relapse in men under sixty years of age who had recently recovered from a first heart attack. This study was conducted by a Research Committee of the Medical Research Council of Great Britain and reported in 1968: 199 men who had recently recovered from a first myocardial infarction were randomly allocated to the experimental group on discharge from four district hospitals in London. The diet for this experimental group was low in saturated fats and contained 85 grams of soybean oil daily; the control patients took their ordinary diets. A high degree of cooperation was achieved. The shortest time in the trial was two years and the longest six and three-quarters years. The test diet lowered the serum cholesterol from a mean initial figure of 272 to 213 mg per 100 ml of serum at six months (a twenty-two-percent decrease), while the level in the control subjects fell from 273 to 259 mgs per 100 ml (a six-percent decline). Sixty-two men on the diet suffered at least one relapse during the period of observation, compared with seventy-four of the control subjects. Forty of the first relapses in the test group were major (i.e., definite reinfarctions or deaths from coronary heart disease), compared with thirty-nine major first relapses among the controls. The total number of men who had a major relapse at any time in the trial was forty-five in the test group and fifty-one in the controls; of these major relapses twenty-five in each group were fatal. None of the differences between the two groups proved significant. Relapses in this study were not related to initial cholesterol level, to change in cholesterol during the trial, nor in any consistent way to observance of the dietary program. There was no evidence from this London trial that the relapse rate in myocardial infarction is materially affected by the unsaturated fat content of the diet used. Why this study is at variance with the others cited is still not evident. The National Heart Foundation of Australia also reported another unsuccessful attempt to obtain secondary prevention by a low-cholesterol, low-saturated-fat diet.

Of the five major attempts to influence favorably the relapse rate in men who had established coronary heart disease, three were apparently successful—but two failed. The reasons for these discrepant results are not clear, but since coronary heart disease is a multifactorial condition we must assume that factors unrelated to the serum cholesterol were more dominant in the London and Australian studies than in the more successful dietary studies in Norway and the United States. Once coronary arteriosclerosis is established to the point where a heart attack has actually occurred it may be too late to expect dietary intervention to reverse the pathologic changes that usually are extensive by this time. Thus, though the results of attempts at secondary prevention seem encouraging, the real test of prophylactic medicine will depend upon the outcome of primary prevention, the ability of the treatment to prevent or delay development of coronary heart disease in normal subjects without preexisting disease of their coronary arteries.

There have now been several studies examining the prophylactic value of cholesterol-reducing diets on the initial occurrence of coronary artery disease—primary prevention. One of the more ambitious of these was recently completed in Finland by Osmo Turpeinen and associates. It included the entire population of two mental hospitals commencing in 1958 and continuing for twelve years. For the first six years the diet in one hospital was changed so that a large part of the milk fat was replaced by an emulsion of soybean oil. Butter and common margarine were replaced by a vegetable margarine high in polyunsaturated fat. In March 1965, just over six years from the initiation of the study, the hospital returned to the normal diet, and the second hospital, which had served as the control population during the first six years, then adopted the experimental diet. The roles of the two hospitals in the experimental design were thus reversed by this crossover arrangement.

The effects of the fat composition of the diet were readily measurable in changes in serum cholesterol concentrations and also in the composition of fat in the adipose tissue. The hospital population receiving the experimental diet showed an average reduction of serum cholesterol of some 50 mgs per 100 ml. The mean of approximately 260 mgs per 100 ml was decreased to a mean of 210 mgs per 100 ml between the two hospitalized populations. With the reversal of diets in 1965 there occurred a corresponding reversal in the serum cholesterol levels.

It has been known since pioneering nutritional studies in domestic animals that the composition of adipose tissue is influenced by the kind of fats in the diet. Small bits of fat tissue were obtained from the subjects in this Finnish study and the fat was analyzed for its composition. Great differences were found in the contents of polyunsaturated fats, which were about two and one-half times higher in the subjects on the experimental diet, while the composition of fats in the adipose tissue of the control group closely resembled that reported for many American and European population groups and contained a proportionately higher fraction of saturated fats. The findings on the composition of adipose tissue are strong evidence that the diets consumed by the two hospital populations did indeed differ in composition of fat as planned and that adherence to the diets was good.

The electrocardiogram was used to detect evidence of new coronary heart disease during this study. Deaths due to coronary occlusion were, of course, also included. There was less new coronary heart disease, by both criteria, in the experimental dietary groups of the two hospitalized populations in each of the two six-year periods covered by the study. The difference was highly significant statistically. Thus the results of a dietary change, which consisted essentially of replacing all milk fat with soybean oil, was followed by a moderate reduction of the serum cholesterol level, a high content of unsaturated fats in adipose tissue, and a considerably lower incidence of new coronary heart disease. Other possible risk factors could not be shown to differ for the two hospital populations, and the crossover design should have eliminated any bias existing in either of the hospital groups.

Though the Finnish study by Dr. Osmo Turpeinen and associates showed a definite decrease in new coronary heart disease in the hospitalized populations fed the low cholesterol diet, there was no difference in overall mortality figures between the control and dietary groups during the twelve years of the study. This had led some to question the significance of the lower incidence of new coronary heart disease resulting from the dietary manipulation. A word on the interpretation of mortality figures is perhaps warranted.

Until the unlikely event that some human being attains immortality, we humans and all animal life are committed to a one to one relationship between life and death. There is no escaping this mortality statistic. Without knowledge of the ages of the individuals in the two hospital populations and in the dietary and control groups at the start of the study and at death the effect on longevity of the diets cannot be assessed. But that was not the question the study was designed to answer. The answer to the question of whether a reduction in the incidence of new coronary heart disease could be produced by the dietary change seems unequivocal, and the causes of death in the dietary and control groups indicated that no other cause of mortality was increased by the low-cholesterol, high-polyunsaturated-fat diets.

Several factors combine to determine the level of cholesterol in the blood: dietary intake, production in the body, and rates of metabolism or excretion. The blood cholesterol is derived both from endogenous synthesis (production in the body) and dietary intake. The relative contribution to the blood cholesterol level of dietary and endogenous sources is complex and variable. Almost every tissue in the body has the capacity to synthesize cholesterol *de novo* from smaller, simpler two-carbon compounds. Only in the case of the liver (which provides more than eighty percent of endogenous cholesterol in the monkey) is the rate of synthesis under dietary control; it is augmented on low cholesterol diets and inhibited by high dietary cholesterol. In man the rate of synthesis of cholesterol in the liver is also inversely related to the dietary intake. Further, the rate of intestinal absorption of cholesterol in man seems limited and is much lower than in the dog, rat, and rabbit. The major and nearly exclusive route by which the body rids itself of cholesterol is via the bowel. This process is dependent in considerable measure on the ability of the liver to convert cholesterol to bile acids.

In addition to rates of intake and output which determine the concentration of cholesterol, not all cholesterol in the blood has an equal likelihood of affecting atheromatous lesions. That cholesterol which is transported in blood in low-density lipoproteins seems to have a particular predilection for arterial walls. This may relate to the protein coat which encases the cholesterol.

The large apparent variability among different individuals in their tolerance to animal fats and cholesterol must also lie in differences in metabolism of these lipids. There are several conditions associated with elevated blood lipids which are hereditary; some of these conditions are associated with the early occurrence of heart attacks. Differences in metabolism rather than diet are responsible here. Not surprisingly, all these factors contribute to the complexity of the relationship between the dietary intake of cholesterol, its blood level, and atherogenesis.

A striking ability to tolerate large quantities of dietary fat and cholesterol is found in the Masai of East Africa. These unique people have milk as their main dietary staple, but they are also fond of fresh cow's blood and the meat of cattle, sheep and goats. When enough milk is available, the average Masai will consume 3 to 5 quarts of whole milk daily, divided usually between two meals. During the dry season, which lasts four to five months, when the supply of milk dwindles, they will bleed the cattle and mix the blood with milk. As compared with standard milk in the United States, their milk contains larger amounts of fat, phospholipids, and cholesterol but lesser amounts of sugar. The protein content is essentially the same. The average daily caloric intake has been estimated to be about 3000 calories, with sixty-six percent of the calories derived from fat. The estimated average daily cholesterol intake is 500 to 2000 mgs per person, which is comparable to that for the average population in the United States. During the dry season, when a thick mixture of milk and blood is drunk and occasionally large amounts of meat are consumed (1814 to 2268 grams at one meal—that is, four to five pounds!), their intake of cholesterol and fat far exceeds that in the average American diet.

In spite of these gross intakes of cholesterol and animal fat it was first observed by George Mann and associates in 1964 that the Masai had low serum cholesterol levels and were free from clinical evidence of atherosclerosis. This striking finding has been recently confirmed by Kurt Biss and his colleagues, who performed ten consecutive autopsies on Masai who had died from accidental causes. The results demonstrated that the Masai's coronary arteries had much thinner walls than those of whites in the United States matched for age and sex. The average serum cholesterol level of Masai over the age of fifteen years was 134 ± 33.5 mg per 100 ml (mean ± standard deviation) and this low value shows no significant increase with increase of age.

The low serum cholesterol levels in the Masai does not represent a failure to absorb ingested cholesterol. They possess, however, an unusually efficient negative feedback system so that the ingested cholesterol inhibits the synthesis of cholesterol in their livers. The body weights of the Masai are much lower than the normal weights for given heights accepted in the United States. Also, their cholesterol pool (the quantity of usable cholesterol in the body) is smaller and turns over more rapidly than ours. These distinct differences between the metabolism of cholesterol in Masai and whites suggests that a genetic trait is responsible. The level of physical activity may, however, be important. It is estimated that they travel some twenty-five miles on foot daily while tending their cattle.

In the United States the serum total cholesterol increases gradually in males from ages eighteen to thirty-three and stabilizes thereafter at about 250 mgs per 100 ml. In women the increase commences some thirteen years later and persists longer to attain values slightly in excess of 250 mgs per 100 ml at age fifty.

By contrast, examination of the serum cholesterol concentration of the villagers of Vilcabamba recently by my colleague, Dr. J. E. Seegmiller, revealed an average serum cholesterol concentration of 148 ± 24 (mean ± standard deviation) mgs per 100 ml for a group of twelve elderly persons ranging from eighty-one to 110 years of age. In fourteen young villagers, nineteen to forty years old, the serum cholesterol averaged 147 ± 27 mgs per 100 ml. Thus, the values are distinctly lower than one would encounter in comparable age groups in this country, and, significantly, there is no increase with age. Values reported recently for serum cholesterol levels of individuals 90 to 140 years of age in Azerbaijan were astoundingly low: 91.8 ± 4.2 milligrams per 100 ml of serum for males and females. Among natives of the Solomon Islands there is also no tendency for the serum cholesterol to rise with age. Thus even our notions of the "normal" or average values for the cholesterol may be biased by the prevalence of high cholesterol diets in our culture.

Atherosclerosis must be regarded as a disease resulting from the interplay of multiple factors, of which cholesterol is an important one. Another important factor is the energy balance of the individual. High levels of physical activity aid the body in the disposition of ingested calories, including atherogenic lipids. Certainly physical activity reduces the incidence and severity of heart attacks. This has been established in several epidemiologic studies. Even the weekend athlete who engages in vigorous physical activity has only one-third the probability of a heart attack compared with his age-matched sedentary neighbors. We don't know, however, whether this beneficial effect of physical exercise is mediated through a lowering of the blood lipids or through an entirely independent action on the circulation.

Thus, the proven or suspected causes of atherosclerosis, the major cause of morbidity and mortality of the aged, include genetic factors, nutrition, and physical activity. But there is ever a suspicion—or often a wishful thought—that nutritional factors other than total calories and the kinds of fats or carbohydrates are involved. Some trace element or vitamin deficiency or excess might be easier to deal with than ingrained habits of overeating and lack of exercise. Epidemiologic studies which have now shown a higher incidence of atherosclerotic heart disease in areas where the water supply is soft than where it is hard reawaken such expectations. It is speculated that the more alkaline, soft water may be corrosive and thus dissolve some metal which causes the atherosclerosis.

The relationship of diet to the occurrence of atherosclerosis seems well documented; diets which promote the accumulation of cholesterol in the body generally increase the likelihood of depositing cholesterol within the walls of arteries and the development of atherosclerosis. It seems probable, however, that injury and pathologic changes in the walls of the arteries must coexist to allow cholesterol to be deposited abnormally in this site. Some recent studies suggest that the initial injury to the walls of arteries may result from a high protein content in a diet insufficient in vitamin B₆. Certain amino acids may damage the fine lining of arteries producing plaques in which cholesterol and fats will deposit in the presence of high concentrations of these substances in the blood. In the absence of elevated blood cholesterol the damage gradually heals.

Diet, Infection, and Cancer

In the case of susceptibility to infections and cancer the role of the diet seems less direct but nevertheless real. Susceptibility to infectious diseases, particularly those of bacterial origin, is generally increased by undernutrition. The pyogenic (pus-forming) bacteria—such as pneumococcus, streptococcus, *Hemophilus influenzae,* and *Pseudomonas pyocyaneus*—are the ones most likely to produce a virulent infection in the malnourished subject. The reason for such susceptibility is the weakening of the immune system in the undernourished individual. The body defends itself against invasion by this group of bacteria through its immune mechanisms. In this instance it is the circulating antibodies produced against these bacteria which are the body's means of defense. The antibodies are produced by specific cells, (small lymphocytes arising from bone marrow and gut-associated lymphoid tissue in mammals) in response to stimulation by antigens (foreign proteins) of the bacteria. But the antibodies are complex proteins, and in the presence of undernutrition or protein deficient diets the production of antibodies is impaired. As a result the host defenses are weak, and the bacterial infection may quickly gain the upper hand. The vulnerability of the poor, the decrepit elderly, and the sickly to infections is the result, at least in part, of deficient antibody formation because of protein deficiency.

Paradoxically, the same protein deficiency may actually diminish the development and spread of cancer in the individual. This has been demonstrated repeatedly in experimental animals and is suggested in man by recent epidemiologic studies. In undernourished animals implanted cancer cells grow less frequently into tumors, and, if once established, tumors spread more slowly than in normally fed animals. The most extensive studies of this type have been performed with inbred strains of mice in which a tumor can be readily passed from one animal to another without the confusing influences of genetic tissue differences. The incidence of spontaneous lung and breast tumors in undernourished mice may reach only sixteen to fifty-five percent of the incidence in well-fed litter mates. The age at which tumors have appeared is almost double, and the average total life span is five times that of normally fed animals.

In one special strain of mice, ninety-five of every 100 animals will spontaneously develop mammary cancer when on an adequate, normal diet. Only five of every 100 animals will develop the cancer if the amount of protein in the diet is markedly reduced. This phenomenon occurs with spontaneous or induced tumors of liver, skin, bone, lymphatic and connective tissue, and bone marrow of mice, rats, and other animals. The decreased incidence of cancers could be produced by diets deficient in calories, in proteins, or in selected essential amino acids— essential because they are required for the synthesis of proteins, but cannot themselves be synthesized by the particular animal species.

Protein deficiency might prevent growth of a tumor simply because of the lack of adequate building blocks to form the tumor. Since tumors grow rapidly, often their need for amino acids with which to make new tumor proteins is great. An inadequate dietary supply might depress growth of the tumor to a larger degree than it depresses the growth of the host. However, the avidity of the growing tumor cells for amino acids is often so great that the tumor will grow at the expense of other body tissues. Thus it appears that other factors associated with general protein deficiency may be important in this resistance to tumor development and growth. One current view is that the immune system is also involved in this phenomenon.

It has been known since before the turn of this century that the immune system produces circulating antibodies which protect the body from bacterial infections, as described. It is only a recent realization that this system is also responsible for self-recognition—that is, the ability to recognize and destroy foreign cells as well as bacteria. This monitoring service is also performed by lymphocytes, but by a different population of lymphocytes than those responsible for producing circulating antibodies which are so essential in combating infections. The lymphocytes which recognize and destroy foreign cells derive from the thymus gland and are often referred to as T-lymphocytes; those responsible for elaborating circulating antibodies are the B-lymphocytes. These T-lymphocytes attack and destroy the foreign intruder and constitute the so-called cellular immune system.

It is thought that cancer cells occur spontaneously and frequently in all of us. However, so long as the T-lymphocytes maintain their normal surveillance function the abnormal cells are promptly destroyed and no harm is done. It is estimated that a child born without a thymus gland—which occurs very rarely—has a probability of developing cancer that is some 10,000 times greater than a normal child of the same age. The lack of the thymus-dependent cellular immune system in such a child is responsible for such an extraordinarily high susceptibility to cancer. Similarly, patients receiving immunosuppressive medicines to prevent rejection of organ transplants or for other indications run a higher risk of developing cancer than normal individuals. Interestingly, the immune system declines in its responsiveness in the later years and this decline corresponds to the greater incidence of cancer in the elderly.

Why should protein deficiency, which interferes with the production of antibodies and thereby increases susceptibility to bacterial infections, enhance the body's resistance to cancer, which is also dependent upon activity of the immune system? The answer seems to lie in the complexity of the immune systems. Apparently the antibody production by B-lymphocytes is diminished more by protein deficiency than is the activity of the T-lymphocytes. There is evidence that antibodies to antigens on the surface of the tumor cells have a blocking effect on the ability of T-lymphocytes to attack and destroy the tumor cells. Protein undernutrition, by preventing the production of such blocking antibodies, leaves the cancer cells vulnerable to destruction by the T-lymphocytes. Cancer grows, according to this view, because one arm of the immune system protects it from destruction by the other. Protein deficiency seems to weaken the arm that protects the cancer.

These new and exciting developments in the relation of the immune systems of the body to cancer and the possible influence of nutrition on this delicate balance await further investigation and clarification. However, we have seen that specific manipulations of the diet may prevent atherosclerotic coronary heart

disease and increase the resistance to cancer, though the necessary manipulation to achieve the latter renders the individual
susceptible to bacterial infection. Humanity may find itself, like
Ulysses, caught between Scylla and Charybdis—an adequate
protein intake necessary to resist infections and a deficient protein
intake to afford resistance to cancer. However, though the time
seems at hand to use dietary measures to prevent heart attacks,
we must await more understanding of cancer and more effective

FIGURE 1

Blocking antibodies may prevent T-lymphocytes from performing
their normal function of recognizing and destroying abnormal
cells in the body. Normally a T-lymphocyte possessing the appropriate specific recognition site would interact with protein
surface antigens on the tumor cells and destroy the latter. If the
tumor surface antigens are, however, covered by circulating
antibodies, then the interaction between T-lymphocytes and
tumor cells is prevented or blocked. Furthermore, tumor cells are
producing new membranes, bits of which may become detached
from the cells. If such a membrane fragment containing a tumor
surface antigen encounters a recognition site on a T-lymphocyte,
it will occupy the recognition site, rendering the T-lymphocyte
impotent in its task of destroying tumor cell.

BLOCKING ANTIBODIES

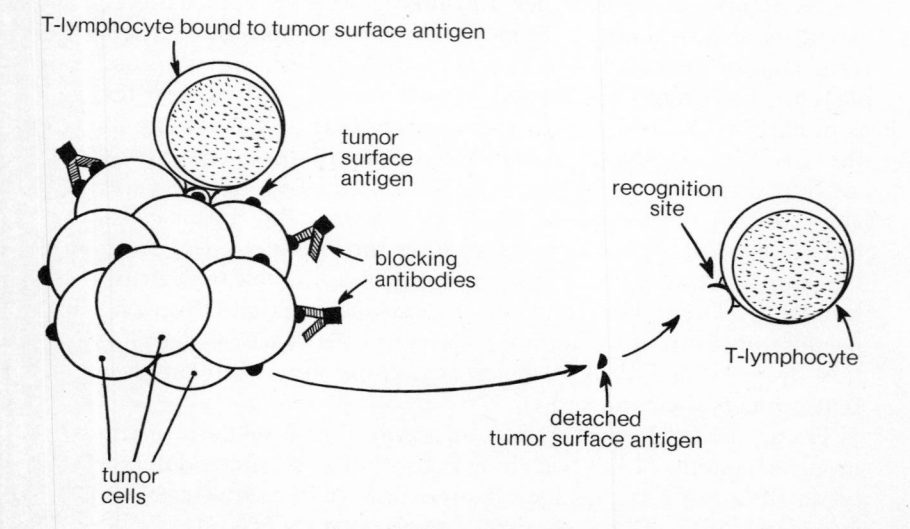

T-lymphocyte bound to tumor surface antigen

tumor
surface
antigen

recognition
site

blocking
antibodies

T-lymphocyte

detached
tumor surface antigen

tumor
cells

means for its control than diet manipulation would seem to afford at present.

Diet may influence the occurrence of cancer in several ways in addition to its potential effect on the immune system. There are some striking geographic variations in the occurrence of specific cancers. The tiny kingdom of Swaziland, the smallest sovereign nation in southern Africa, has an inordinately high incidence of cancer of the liver. In the United States primary cancer of the liver is relatively rare, but in other parts of Africa, as well as in Swaziland, it is very prevalent. The villain seems to be a toxin, "aflatoxin," produced by a common mold, *Aspergillus flavus*. This mold has a predilection for peanuts and some grains, which if stored or processed under humid conditions may provide favorable conditions for growth of the mold. When ingested in large amounts this aflatoxin may produce massive necrosis of the liver, but in small amounts it can cause liver cancer. Proper curing and storing of peanuts can largely abolish this very lethal cancer.

In recent years there has been a rapid increase in the United States of cancer of the colon and rectum. After skin cancer it is now the most common cancer in the United States, topping in incidence both lung and breast cancer, and it is second only to lung cancer in the number of cancer deaths. It is estimated that 99,350 Americans will develop the malignancy next year, which will be an increase of 15.6 percent in five years. The colon–rectal cancer rate has climbed to 46.8 per 100,000 Americans from forty-three per 100,000 in 1968 and 39.3 per 100,000 in 1947. In other parts of the world cancer of the colon and rectum is rare. In Japan and Chile cancer of the large bowel is uncommon, but cancer of the stomach, which has largely disappeared in the United States over the past twenty to thirty years, is very prevalent. These curious patterns of distribution are not genetically determined. Japanese who have migrated to Hawaii in the 1920s and 1930s and have adopted American eating habits are showing a higher incidence of colonic cancer than encountered in Japan, though still less than that characteristic of the United States population.

The linking of colon–rectal cancer with the diet is, at the moment, largely statistical, but some interesting speculations have been presented. One view links cancer of the large bowel to consumption of beef. Thus the incidence of this cancer is highest in Scotland and Denmark and other beef-eating countries, but low where vegetables and grains constitute the main staples of the diet. The suggestion that beef is specifically involved comes indirectly from epidemiologic studies pursued by Drs. John W. Berg and William Haenszel at the National Cancer Institute. They point out that in Scotland and Denmark cancer of the large bowel afflicts rural rather than urban populations as is the case elsewhere. These rural areas are the beef-raising and beef-eating districts, especially Aberdeen and its neighbors. Moreover, while the Scots consume less meat than any part of England, they eat more beef than the English and have a proportionately higher mortality rate from bowel cancer.

Others have attributed the relationship to the ingestion of animal fats and cholesterol which would increase the secretion of bile acids into the bowel. The steroid molecules of the bile might then undergo bacterial alteration to carcinogens in the bowel. Many chemical carcinogens are cyclic hydrocarbons with a basic structure similar to that of cholesterol. This view has been amplified by the British surgeon and epidemiologist, Dr. Denis Burkitt. He observed that among the Bantu of Africa the high content of unrefined grains in the diet leads to a rapid transit time of food through the intestines. The rural African, Burkitt points out, continues to eat a large amount of unrefined cereals, while European and American consumption of whole wheat flour, bran, and other vegetable roughage has dropped to a fifth or tenth of what it was in 1900. He theorizes that whatever cancer-causing substances may be present in food waste will be in contact with the colon for a longer time among Westerners than among Africans. As mentioned, slow passage through the bowel would allow bacterial alteration of bile acids and other lipids with formation of possible carcinogens which also would have longer contact with the lining of the colon.

When I was an intern thirty years ago there were always several cases of cancer of the stomach in the hospital. The differential diagnosis between benign peptic ulceration and cancerous ulceration of the stomach was one of the frequent problems with which we dealt. Today cancer of the stomach is unusual in the United States but prevalent in Japan. Japanese who migrated to California have a lower incidence of this cancer, especially if they are second-generation Japanese born in the United States. Chinese are susceptible to cancer of the nasopharynx so long as they live in China. Many also have migrated to California; by the second and third generations their diets differ little from that of other Americans. The incidence of cancer of the nose and throat then declines. Esophageal cancer shows a curious geographic distribution. While fortunately rare in the United States, it occurs in the Transkei area of the Republic of South Africa and in parts of Iran more frequently than anywhere else in the world and has reached almost epidemic proportions among the natives of these regions. There have been many speculations but no satisfactory explanation as to what it is in habits and diet that produces these curious geographic oddities in the prevalence or absence of cancer.

The role of the diet in sustaining optimal health is an important one. Undoubtedly further research will reveal individual needs not only for the major dietary constituents—proteins, lipids, and carbohydrates—but also for vitamins and trace elements about which we know very little at present. The hope that some dietary factor will do for humans what royal jelly does for bees is oft-reborn. By selecting one larva from thousands of genetically identical larvae and feeding it continuously on royal jelly, a queen bee is created. Her life span is ten fold—or greater—than that of her sisters destined to become short-lived workers. Surely this represents the ultimate in the nutritional extension of the life span!

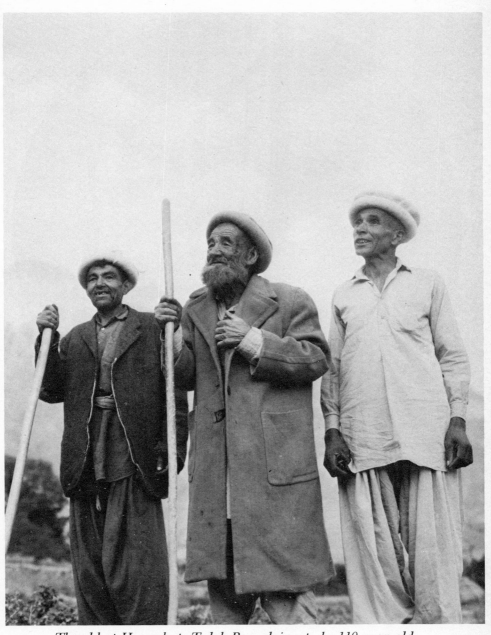

The oldest Hunzukut, Tulah Beg, claims to be 110 years old.
He stands between his two sons, Nigar Shah, seventy-five, and
Sagi Ali, seventy.

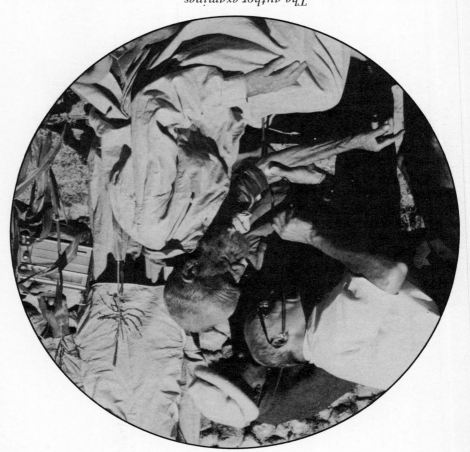

*The author examines
Tulah Beg, and finds
him in good condition.*

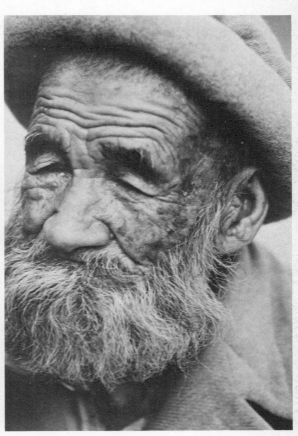

A portrait of Tulah Beg.

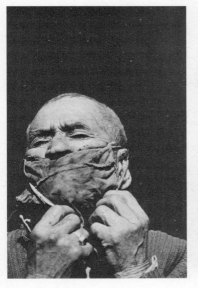

Gul Baig, age ninety-five, dyes his beard red with henna.

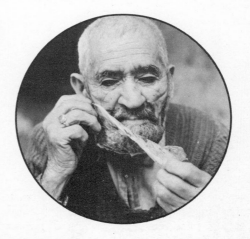

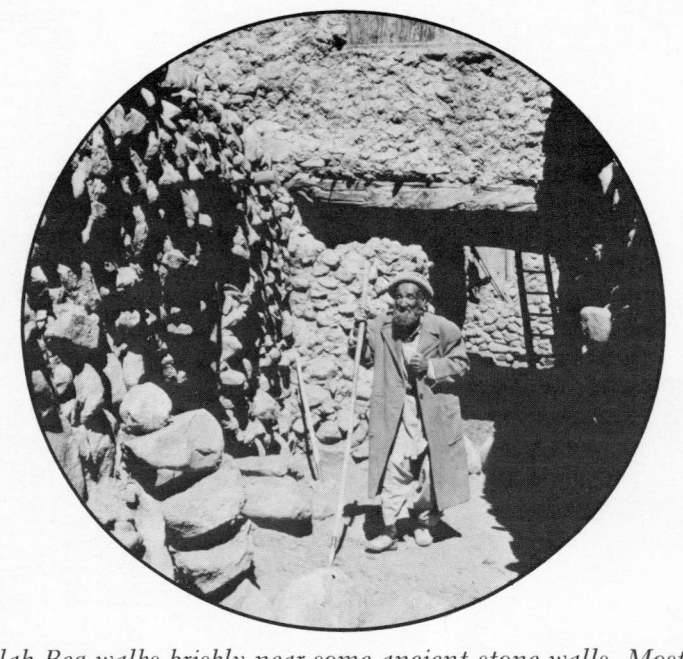

Tulah Beg walks briskly near some ancient stone walls. Most of the buildings are made of stones.

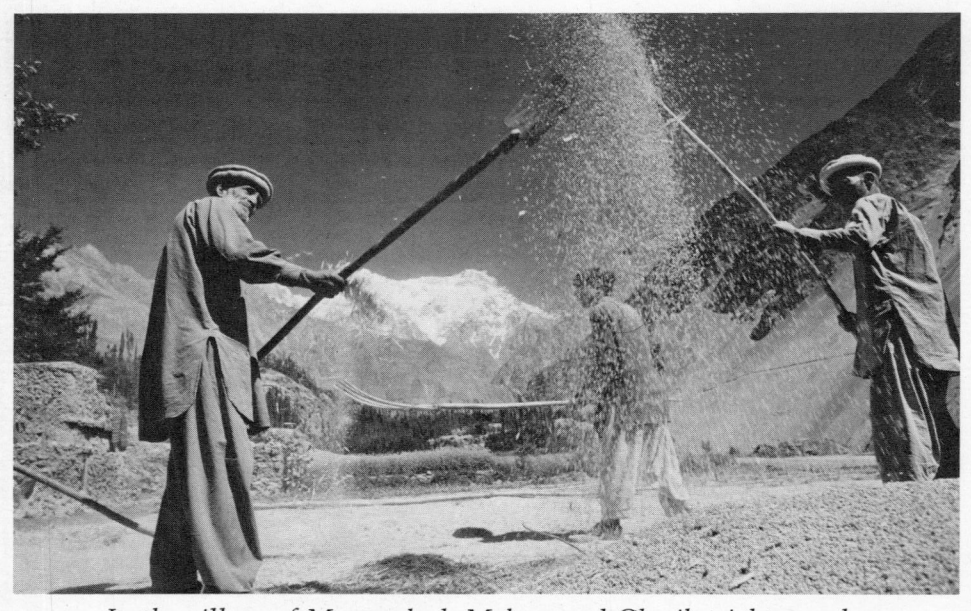

In the village of Murtazabad, Mohammed Ghraib, eighty, and Ibrahim Shah, seventy-five, winnow wheat. In the background is Mt. Ultar.

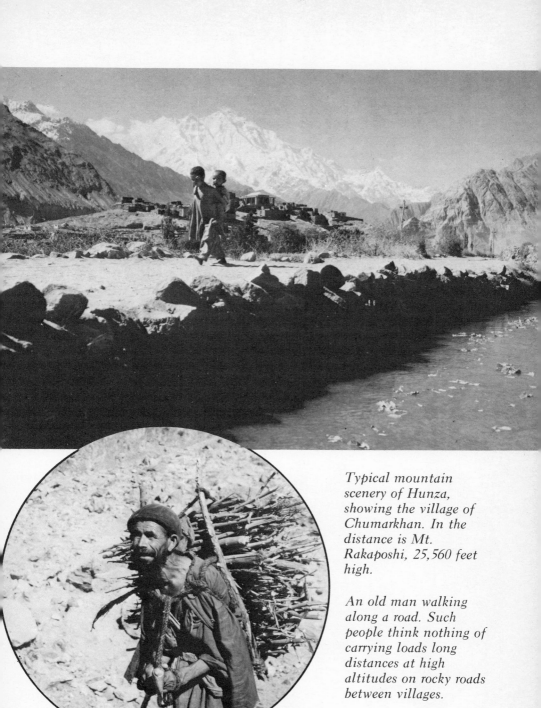

Typical mountain scenery of Hunza, showing the village of Chumarkhan. In the distance is Mt. Rakaposhi, 25,560 feet high.

An old man walking along a road. Such people think nothing of carrying loads long distances at high altitudes on rocky roads between villages.

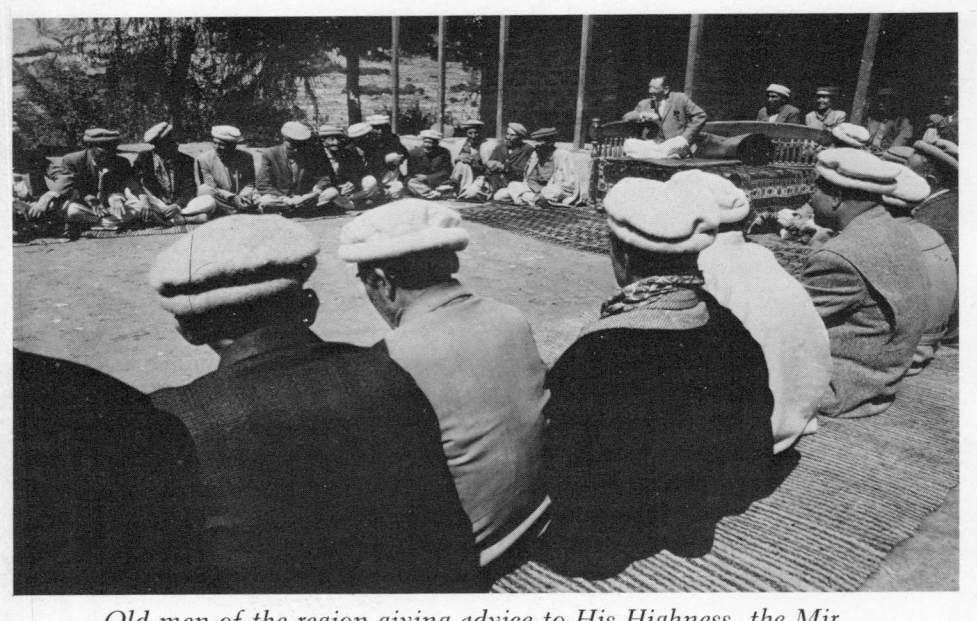

Old men of the region giving advice to His Highness, the Mir, leader of the Hunzas.

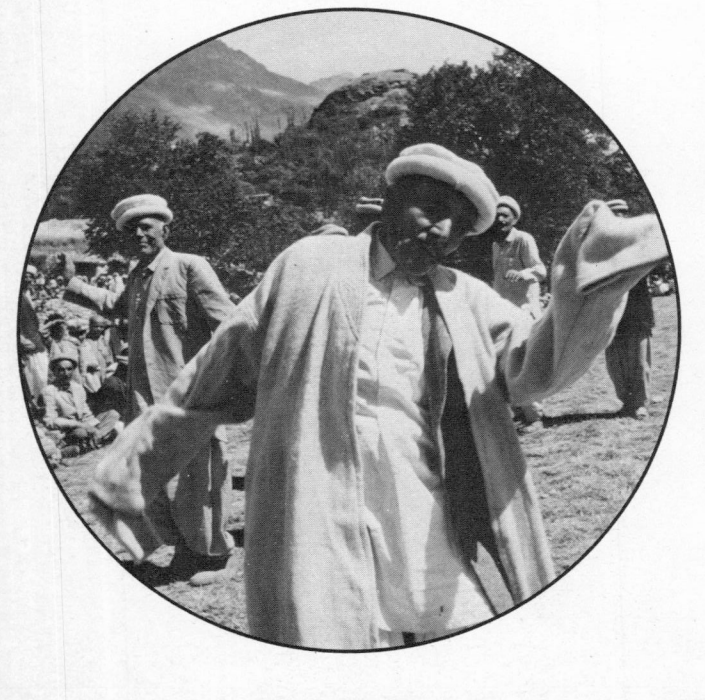

Ninety-nine-year-old Kabul Hyat leads a state dance in celebration of the crown prince's marriage festivities.

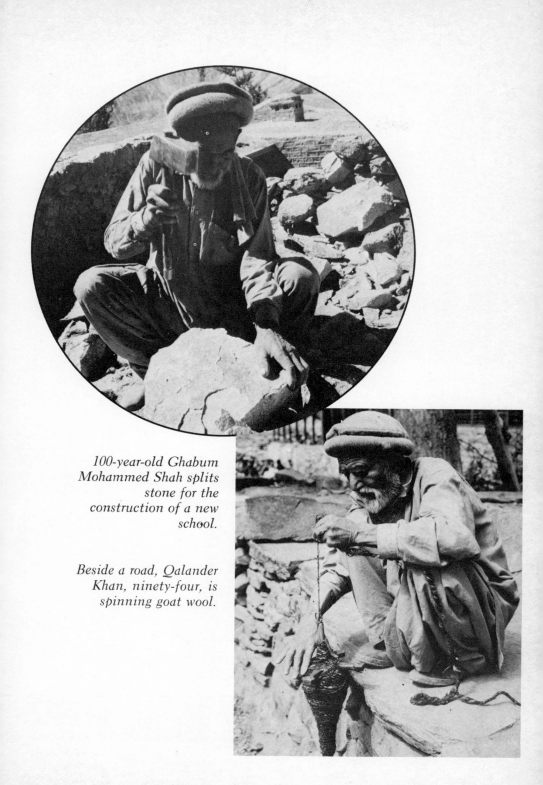

100-year-old Ghabum Mohammed Shah splits stone for the construction of a new school.

Beside a road, Qalander Khan, ninety-four, is spinning goat wool.

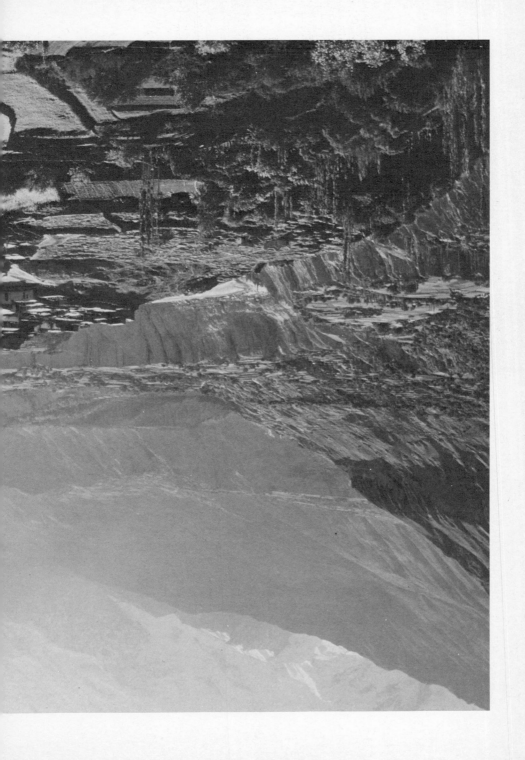

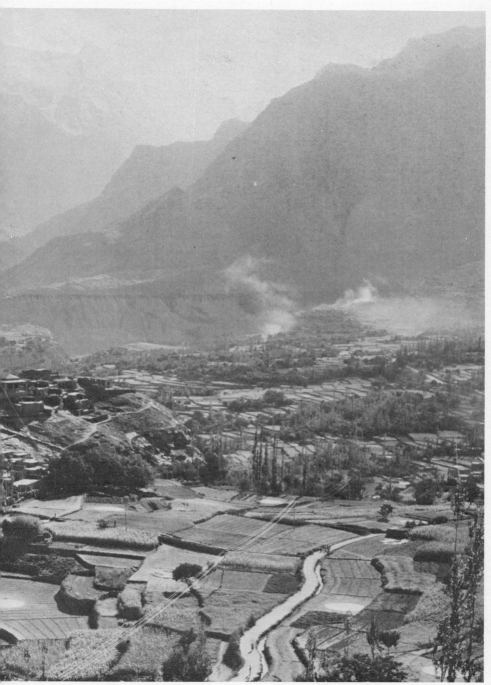

An overview of the valley of Hunza. Across the Hunza River is Nagir. Mt. Rakaposhi is in the distance.

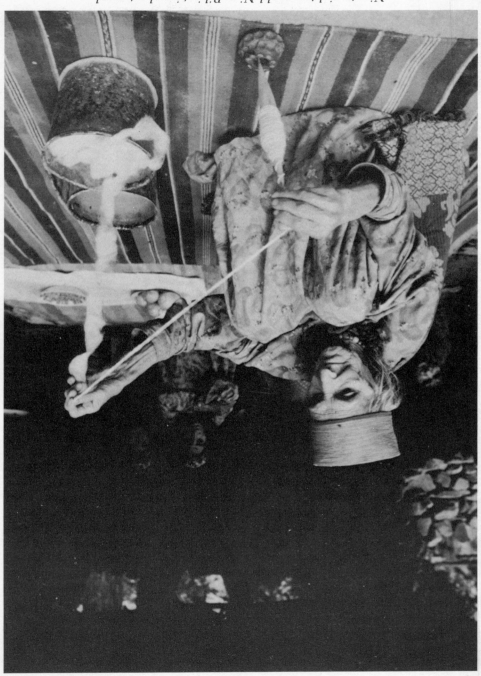

Ninety-eight-year-old Niay Bibi spins sheep wool.

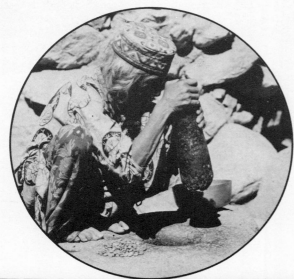

Seventy-five-year-old Dault Bibi, daughter of ninety-five-year-old Niay, is crushing apricot stones to make oil.

Ninety-year-old Begum Murad Shah sorting dried apricots on the rooftop of her house. In the background is Mt. Rakaposhi.

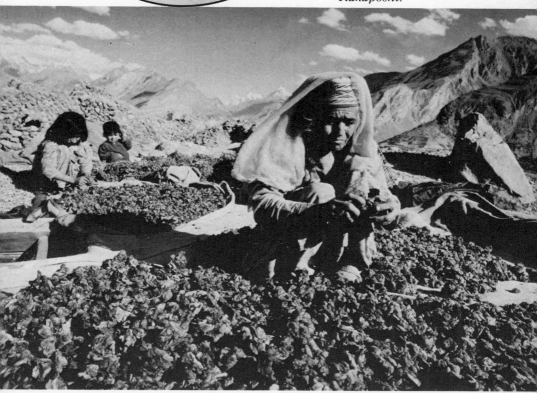

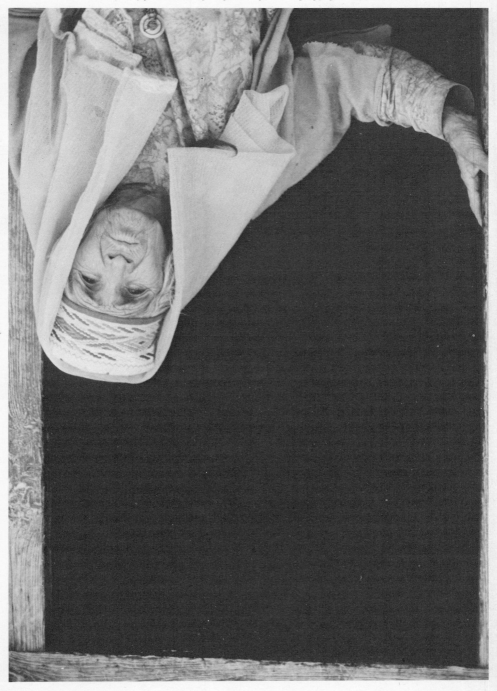
Begum Murad Shah stands in the doorway of her house.
She is wearing a typical costume of the region.

PHYSICAL ACTIVITY

Those who think they have not time for bodily exercise will sooner or later have to find time for illness.

Edward Stanley, Earl of Derby (1826–1893), "The Conduct of Life," (address at Liverpool College, December 20, 1873)

listened to Dr. David Kakiashvili as we bumped together in the rear seat of our car. We drove into the countryside to a remote collective farm where many old people reportedly lived. "Why do people in the small mountain villages tolerate heart attacks much better than their urbanized relatives?" he asked. Getting no response from me, he continued, "The constant physical activity required of them develops the function of their hearts and lungs so that the oxygen supply to their hearts is much superior to that in city dwellers. Thus the collateral circulation is well developed and heart attacks are better tolerated."

Dr. Kakiashvili had been studying gerontology in the Caucasus for twelve years when I met him. He is convinced that the continuous and mandatory, if involuntary, exercise to which the mountain dwellers are subjected is a major factor in their longevity. He has studied the function of heart and lungs of these old people in detail, using modern sophisticated investigative techniques, and he finds that the old people have many types of cardiovascular diseases. He found evidence of frequent heart attacks, but these were apparently "silent" and not accompanied by the usual clinical symptoms in most instances.

I had gone through several stages in my thinking regarding the relationship of the mountainous terrain in the three places I visited and the longevity of the people there. At first I speculated that the remoteness of the regions protected these people from the ravages of infectious diseases from the surrounding populations. Even though these communities may have been off the main path of the major scourges of mankind, still there was a considerable number of infectious diseases among them, and most varieties seemed to be represented. Then I wondered if, because of the remoteness of their habitat, a small group of individuals with genes favorable to a long life had avoided mating with individuals having a lesser genetic endowment. It is thought that there are no genes for longevity—only genes that may increase the probability of contracting or developing some fatal illness. A group of individuals lacking such "bad" genes might procreate and in time express their genetic tendency toward longevity. Inbreeding generally causes deterioration of the stock, but a long-lived product in these special situations seemed a possibility. Such a thesis might be appropriate for Vilcabamba and even Hunza but the multiple ethnic backgrounds of the old people in the Caucasus seem a contradiction.

Physical factors associated with altitude were considered. Adaptation of the cardiovascular system to altitude at first seemed a possibility, but altitudes of 2000 to 6000 feet that were involved do not require specific adaptation or at most very minimal adaptation. Purity of the air in these remote areas may be a factor. Though environmental pollution undoubtedly can be a negative factor, its absence can hardly be a positive factor in unusual longevity. The incidence of cosmic rays or other ionizing radiation may be unusual in these three areas but there is no factual basis for this supposition or others relating altitude and isolation to longevity.

Finally, I came to the same conclusion as Dr. Kakiashvili—that the inevitable necessity for a high level of physical fitness conditioned by the steep terrain was very important. Simply to get through the day's chores required a great deal of physical exertion. No one sits at a desk or rides to and from work. The simple task of walking from one dwelling to the next or from a village down to the surrounding fields and back left us huffing and puffing, but even the oldest natives negotiated these steep slopes agilely. Their traditional farming and household practices demand heavy physical work; throughout their lives, men and women are constantly busy. Superimposed on the usual effort of farming are the added demands resulting from the mountainous terrain. Simply traversing the hills by foot during the course of the day's activities will sustain a high degree of cardiovascular fitness.

A striking difference between our bodies and a high-quality mechanical device such as a bicycle or automobile is that we improve with usage, while the mechanical device can only deteriorate from wear and tear. As long as we are in good health and the activity not too violent, our bodies will respond positively to the challenge. It is common experience that muscles enlarge and strengthen with repeated exercise. This results from an increase in the size and contractile force of individual muscle cells rather than from an increase in the number of muscle cells. Exercise increases muscle mass largely through an increase in the size of each cell. This is accompanied by an increase in protein content of the muscle. The contractile fibrils of the muscle increase in number and they contract more efficiently— i.e., the tension developed or the work done on contracting increases with exercise and the energy cost per unit of work performed decreases.

The adaptive response to exercise affects not only the skeletal muscles in arms, legs, back, etc., which are directly involved in the exercise activity. Muscles of respiration work harder as the exercise stimulates an increased depth and rate of breathing. But the heart, which is also a muscle, contracts more vigorously and more rapidly. An increase in pulse rate and in the volume of blood ejected by the heart with each beat is the response of this organ to the increased blood supply needed by the working muscles during exercise. With repeated exercises the heart is able to do its job more efficiently requiring a lesser increase in pulse rate and in the volume of blood pumped per unit of time for a given degree of physical activity.

Exercise improves the circulation to nearly all parts of the body. Circulation is increased to the brain as well as to the heart and skeletal muscles. Recently it has been asserted that increase in the oxygen supply to the brain will actually improve thinking. In a resting sedentary individual, however, the blood supplied to the brain contains more oxygen than the brain is able to extract. It is difficult to see how a further excess of a constituent that is normally not a rate-limiting factor in cerebral function would enhance that function. It may, nevertheless, be that the sense of well-being that the exercising individual enjoys is likely to increase his self-confidence and as a result improve both social and intellectual effectiveness.

An organ that throughout life is continually remodeling to the stresses put upon it by exercise is the skeleton, our bony scaffolding. A continuous process of building and demolition goes on in our bones. New bone is laid down to provide increased strength at points of stress, while unstressed bone is reabsorbed. This keeps the mass and strength of our bones commensurate with their use. Of course, too sudden a stress on a bone may result in its fracture. However, degrees of stress, short of creating a fracture, will lead to a heightened deposition of new bone and decrease in reabsorption of bone locally to result in a marked increase in the strength of the bone.

Osteoporosis is a condition all too common in our elderly. It is literally an increased porosity of the bones. Both the mineral content—the calcium salts that make the bones hard and strong—and the collagen and cartilage, which are the matrix in which the calcium salts are deposited, diminish. Bones become thin, less dense, and more fragile. They become very vulnerable to fracture with only slight trauma. The fracture of the head of the femur, hip fracture, or collapse of the body of a vertebra, which may result in the elderly from what appears to be a rather trivial fall, is the consequence of osteoporosis.

In the Caucasian village of Duripshi we drove with Markhti Tarkhil, age 104, on foot down a steep dirt road to the river below. It proved to be a difficult and rough descent, but Markhti moved so quickly and agilely over the rocks and down the river bank that I had difficulty keeping up with him. I ran, jumped, and slithered down the rocks to keep beside him, frightened at what might happen were he to stumble and fall. Knowing how fragile the bones of most of our old people are, I had terrifying visions of picking up the pieces were Markhti to trip. Fortunately no such mishap occurred and Markhti reached the bottom of the hill ahead of me.

Later I asked the Russian doctors there how often the old people suffer fractures. They shrugged and claimed it just didn't happen. The constant physical activity keeps the balance between bone formation and destruction such that the bones of these vigorous elders remain mineralized, dense, and strong. With inactivity at any age our bones lose their calcium salts and become thin and fragile, just as our muscles atrophy and become smaller and weaker with disuse. In our aged, inactivity together with a general tendency toward reduced tissue mass, may result in such a loss of bone mass that slight trauma suffices to cause fractures. A hip fracture with the resultant immobilization in bed and the complications which all too often follow may prove the terminal event. In spite of efforts with hormones, vitamin D and high intakes of calcium and phosphorus the treatment of osteoporosis in our old people has resisted cure. Continued physical exertion remains the most potent preventive measure against this debility.

Recent studies on our astronauts by a team of investigators from our National Institutes of Health have clearly demonstrated that lack of stress on the skeletal system is a major hazard to space flight. They found that, under the conditions of weightlessness that exist during interplanetary flight, even strictly imposed regimens of exercise were unable to prevent rapid dissolution of bone with a resultant large outpouring of calcium from the skeleton. Prolonged exposure to weightless conditions would not only create the risk of fractures from weakening and thinning of bones, but the rate of dissolution of the bones may exceed the body's ability to excrete the calcium, with the resultant abnormal precipitation of calcium phosphate in body tissues. The kidneys are particularly vulnerable to damage from the precipitation of calcium salts either as stones obstructing the urinary passageways or as finer deposits of calcium salts within the substance of the kidney which interfere with the function of these important organs.

Although exercise undoubtedly benefits the musculoskeletal system, it is the circulation which is the real beneficiary of regular exercise. Many doctors have recommended physical exercise as a prophylactic against arteriosclerosis and coronary disease. There is a classic British study which compared the incidence of heart attacks among postal workers in London. Those who carried the mail bags and delivered the mail had a lower total incidence of myocardial infarction and a lesser mortality and morbidity than did their sedentary colleagues working at desk jobs in the post office. The case-fatality was a third in the postmen (fifty-one of 171), compared with almost one-half of the telephonists, executives, and clerks (seventy of 143).

Another part of the same study compared the incidence of heart attacks among London bus drivers with that among an age-matched group of conductors on the buses. The latter, who continually move up and down the double-decker buses collecting the fares, suffered a lesser incidence and mortality from heart attacks than did the sedentary drivers. Here the emotional stress of driving through the London traffic may have been a factor weighted also against the bus drivers. In both groups studied the physically active group had less coronary heart disease; and what disease they did have was less severe.

J. N. Morris, who conducted these studies, was responsible for a large postmortem study in Great Britain as well. This national necropsy survey compared the incidence at postmortem examination of changes in the heart which could be attributed to coronary heart disease in those whose employment involved heavy physical work and in those whose work was sedentary. It was found that physical activity is a real protection against coronary heart disease. Men in physically active jobs have less coronary heart disease during middle age, what disease they have is less severe, and they develop it later than men in physically inactive jobs. The hearts of sedentary and light workers showed the pathology of the hearts of heavy workers ten to fifteen years older.

A group of physicians which has been especially interested in physical fitness has organized the American Medical Joggers Association. It has followed the obituary notices of all physicians dying in this country, and claims not to have found a single case of coronary heart disease among marathon runners. Its view is that such exercise protects the heart from coronary heart disease. It regards endurance exercises rather than competitive speed racing as the most beneficial form. Thus it advises that the jogger not increase his speed when he can easily accomplish a two-mile jog but rather add another mile to his exercise program. This kind of exercise they believe is beneficial and can be done at any age, provided that one begins gradually.

Competitive, very strenuous exercises which place a sudden very large stress on our hearts, on the other hand, may be harmful. Such strenuous exertion may create an oxygen deficit in active muscles, including the heart, which is also a muscle. An oxygen debt occurs during exercise whenever the oxygen required to meet the energy needs of muscle contraction exceeds the rate of delivery of oxygen by the blood to the contracting muscle. Trained athletes who compete in the 100-yard dash generally do not breathe during the intense burst of activity. They may acquire a considerable oxygen deficit during a race. Marathon runners, on the other hand, maintain a pace which allows essentially complete oxidation of the glucose and fats which provide the energy for their muscles.

In the presence of intense exercise and an oxygen deficit the manner by which the muscles burn sugars and fats changes. Muscles fall back on a more primitive form of energy metabolism called "glycolysis." During glycolysis, glucose, the sugar of our body, is only partially oxidized and is split into two molecules of lactic acid. This releases only one-eighteenth the energy that can be provided by the complete oxidation of glucose to carbon dioxide and water. The lactic acid, however, accumulates and produces a degree of acidosis which is proportional to the magnitude of the oxygen lack. A decreased supply of energy to the heart just at a time when its energy requirements are greatest and the acidic condition produced by the lactic acid may impair the function of the heart muscle.

If the blood vessels to the heart are narrowed by atherosclerosis the supply of blood to the heart muscle may be borderline—just sufficient to bring enough oxygen to provide its normal needs at rest. With only slight exertion, or with increased heart rate, the delivery of oxygen may quickly become inadequate to meet the needs of the heart muscle. Although the normal heart can tolerate such brief bouts of relative oxygen deficit, when the coronary arteries are diseased, angina pectoris (a squeezing discomfort in the midchest often elicited by exercise or emotion and which may signify insufficient blood flow to the heart muscle), heart failure, or even a heart attack may be precipitated by such sudden exertion. The diminished energy available within the muscle cells and the effects of lactic acid accumulating in the heart muscle may weaken its contractions, interfere with con-duction of impulses within the heart muscle which is essential for the coordinated contraction of the heart, and cause irregularities of the pulse rate or fatal arrest of the heart.

No adequate data exist on which to decide what kinds of exercise are most beneficial in conditioning the heart and lungs to supply oxygen optimally to the body. However, common sense would seem to favor repetitive endurance exercises (such as long walks, jogging, slow swimming, bicycle riding), carried to the point of stressing the heart and lungs mildly. Evidence of such stress is noted by the subjective sense of shortness of breath. This feeling is noted when the exchange of air with each breath approaches the vital capacity of the lungs. At rest we exchange only some 400 to 600 cubic centimeters of air with each breath, whereas with a maximal inspiration following a complete expira-tion our lungs may accommodate 3000 to 5000 cc. of air (vital capacity). When we become short of breath from exercise the volume of air exchanged with each breath approaches the vital capacity.

Exercise stress also manifests itself by an acceleration of the heart rate. In order to deliver more oxygen to the exercising muscles the output of the heart increases and the circulation of blood is enhanced. This is accomplished by a greater volume of blood pumped with each contraction of the heart and also by an increased rate of the heartbeat or pulse. A pulse rate increasing from a resting level of 60 to 75 up to 120 beats per minute represents an adequate stress to the heart.

In the present decade there has been an increased interest in exercise as a form of therapy for the heart which is affected by angina pectoris or which has sustained one or more infarctions. The physiologic basis of the favorable clinical effects of any intervention such as exercise is dependent upon improving the balance between the supply of oxygen to the heart muscle and the needs of the heart muscle for oxygen. Because ischemia (inadequate blood supply) occurs when the oxygen consumption exceeds the capacity of the diseased coronary arteries to deliver oxygen, the success of all forms of treatment depends on a favorable alteration of this balance; either the capacity of the coronary system to deliver blood to the ischemic regions of the heart muscle must be improved or the demand of the heart muscle for oxygen must be reduced. It may not, therefore, be immediately apparent why exercise which increases the work of the heart should be useful therapeutically when the coronary vessels are already diseased.

Nevertheless, it is now well established that physical training increases the exercise tolerance and performance of individuals with ischemic heart disease. The studies have generally indicated a more efficient circulatory response to exercise as a result of physical training. That is, the demands of the heart muscle for any given level of exercise decrease with physical training. This allows the individual an increased level of exercise before the supply of oxygen limits further exertion. Thus, a major effect of training is an increase in exercise capacity resulting in a more efficient circulatory response to exercise. This is accomplished through several adjustments.

First, the physically trained person will have a slower heart rate at rest and experience a lesser increase in pulse rate for a given level of exercise or exertion than an untrained individual. The heart receives the nutrient blood supply to its muscle during diastole—that is, in the period of relaxation between contractions. The time devoted to contraction of the heart muscle, systole, is short and relatively constant and independent of the heart rate. Thus a slow heart rate indicates proportionately longer diastoles and hence a longer time for blood to flow through the coronary arteries to nurture the heart muscle. The effect of physical training to slow the heart rate will therefore provide a longer time for and an improved delivery of oxygen to the contracting muscle. This is one factor in the increased efficiency of the circulation induced by physical training.

Another positive effect of training is a lowering of blood

pressure. The increased blood flow to the exercising muscles in part results from a dilatation of the blood vessels in the muscle. The heat generated by the exercise is largely dissipated through the skin. Dilation of the blood vessels in the skin thus also accompanies exercise. But skin and muscles make up the major mass of the body and dilation of their blood vessels reduces blood pressure. This means that the circulating blood encounters a low resistance, and therefore it takes less effort on the part of the heart to force the blood through the vessels. The reactivity of the small arteries in skin and muscle improves with training; and thus the heart is able to supply the requisite blood flow to the body at a lower cost in its own oxygen needs. Thus, again training has improved the balance of myocardial oxygen supply for a given level of oxygen needs by the heart and the exercising muscles.

In the normal heart the coronary blood vessels will dilate to provide an increased supply of blood to the heart muscle during exertion. Whether such an enhanced blood flow can occur with physical training in narrowed, atherosclerotic diseased coronary vessels is not so clearly demonstrated. However, it does appear that with prolonged periods of gradually increasing physical activity even the ischemic heart muscle may benefit by an increased delivery of oxygen. Whether this is the result of the growth of new blood vessels into the ischemic area or a clearing of the arteriosclerotic process within the diseased coronary vessels to accommodate an increased blood flow to the ischemic area is still not proven.

Regular vigorous, but not too strenuous or exhausting, exercise thus will not only protect the heart from the insult of coronary atherosclerosis but will increase exercise capability in patients who unfortunately have acquired coronary disease. Training not only reduces the oxygen demands of the heart for a given level of exertion but also increases the blood flow to the heart muscle in the normal subject and most likely in the patient with ischemic heart disease.

Another potentially important effect of exercise is to increase the ability of the blood to dissolve blood clots. The cause of the deposition of cholesterol, calcium salts, blood clots and connective tissue in the walls of arteries, which narrows the caliber of blood vessels and renders them rigid is not yet known. The initial injury seems to involve the smooth muscle cells in the walls of the blood vessels, but later the cells lining the blood vessels as well are affected. The plaques which are formed may project into the opening of the artery, be dislodged and carried away by the flowing blood to obstruct some smaller blood vessel into which the larger artery branches.

One hypothesis for the development of atherosclerosis is the so-called thrombogenic theory according to which atherosclerotic plaques originate as a result of fibrin deposits on the inner lining of the affected artery. Fibrin is the protein in blood which forms the matrix in which the red blood cells and other constituents of the blood are enmeshed in the formation of a blood clot. Recently, it has been suggested that tissues are normally undergoing injury and repair, and with this there may be a balance between deposition and solution of fibrin in any blood vessel. An imbalance favoring clot formation would occur if the process of solution of fibrin were impaired. This might lead to persistence of fibrin deposits at the inner surface of a vessel, and ultimately degeneration of the vessel wall at this site with appearance of an atherosclerotic plaque.

Some reduction in fibrinolytic activity (the ability of blood to dissolve fibrin) has been found in association with atherosclerosis. There is still considerable uncertainty whether the deposition of fibrin is an initial step in the development of atherosclerotic changes in a vessel or a late, secondary event taking place on an already damaged inner surface of blood vessels. Most would subscribe to the latter view. Nevertheless, fibrin is a regular but abnormal constituent within the atherosclerotic plaques. Exercise of a vigorous nature is effective in increasing fibrinolytic activity of blood and may in this manner also protect against the development of atherosclerosis.

Undoubtedly the best use of exercise is prophylactic. A recent study reported in *Lancet*, an important British medical journal, showed that even the "weekend" athlete is benefitted prophylactically. Adult males who devoted some portion of their weekends to vigorous exercise (reaching peaks of expenditure of energy of $7^{1}/_{2}$ calories per minute) suffered only one-third the incidence of coronary heart disease of their age-matched sedentary neighbors. Jogging, bicycling, swimming, tennis, heavy work such as digging, and other such activities qualify as adequate forms of exercise to produce this beneficial effect.

In Evans County, Georgia, U.S.A., an astute and enterprising general practitioner, Curtis Hames, M.D., had observed a high incidence of coronary heart disease among his white male patients but few instances of heart attacks among black males. A study reported by J. C. Cassel of essentially all the adults over forty years of age and of half of those between fifteen and thirty-nine years, over an eighteen-month period from 1960 to 1962, confirmed Dr. Hames's observation. Ninety-one percent of the population was reexamined in similar fashion between 1967 and 1969.

As a result of these extensive observations three groups of men could be identified with respect to incidence of coronary heart disease. Two groups, white sharecroppers and black men, had less than half the incidence of coronary heart disease of the third group, all other white men. The incidence of heart attacks in the latter group of white nonfarmers is among the highest in the country. It was the level of physical activity required by the blacks and white sharecroppers which largely protected these two groups from coronary artery disease. Most other risk factors measured—namely, blood pressure, serum cholesterol level, cigarette smoking, body weight, and diet—could not account for the differences.

During my last few days in Abkhasia I had learned that one old man from the mountain village of Hopee was spending the summer as usual with his goats in the high alpine pastures. Since I was told he was 106 years old I decided that I must see him in that setting and learn at first hand the physical exertion involved in his daily activities. I started early one morning with three companions. The trail was muddy, slippery, and so steep that we were often climbing rather than hiking; two of our party, in fact, gave up about one-third of the way and headed back downhill. It was only the thought of how dreadful the steep slippery descent would be that kept me going up with my young guide, a local schoolmaster.

After about six hours of climbing we came out of the woods onto a grassy slope and found Kosta Kashig, who claimed to be 106 years old. He lived with two men and a boy as companions in an open lean-to built of wood saplings covered with plastic sheet for a roof and with goatskins covering the floor. Their outdoor kitchen consisted of an iron cauldron suspended over an open fire from the ridge pole at the front of their lean-to. In it they cooked *abusta*, a thick corn meal mush, which they stirred with a large wooden spoon and ate with red peppers. The remainder of their diet was obtained from their goats and included soured milk, cheese, and some meat.

Since my interpreter had dropped out during the climb,

interrogation of Kosta was difficult, but I concluded he was ninety rather than 106. Whichever is correct, however, to be able to spend four months of the year bounding over the hillside from dawn until dusk in pursuit of his agile goats seemed remarkable enough.

My own elation over getting up to the high pasture land was quelled when I was informed, after I had returned exhausted to the village below, that the old man made the same trek in just half the time it took me.

Rest is the counterpart of physical activity and just as essential for good health. It is during rest and sleep that the vegetative functions of our bodies restore and replenish damage from the stresses of our activities. The pattern of rest and the amount of sleep required by the elderly was very variable.

In documenting the daily routine of a large group of Georgians eighty years of age and over, Professor Pitzkhelauri found ample time allotted for rest. His figures indicate some ten hours for sleep at night—to bed at 9 to 10 P.M. and up at 8 to 9 A.M. in the winter and an hour later to bed but an hour earlier up in the mornings during spring and summer. A two- to three-hour siesta in the midafternoon (3 to 5 or 4 to 7 P.M.) was common. The main meal of the day tended to be from two to four P.M. with a supper in the evening, 6 to 7:30 P.M. From supper to bedtime was devoted to a variety of relaxing family activities: playing with grandchildren, listening to radio, watching television or reading newspapers, visiting friends and relatives, playing musical instruments or singing. This left five hours in the winter and eight hours during spring and summer for household chores and work on the farm.

Many individuals note that their nocturnal sleep requirements may decrease with advanced age. Elderly patients often complain of wakefulness and inability to sleep through the night. The disruption of the normal sleep pattern is often accompanied by the need for an afternoon nap which may in turn reduce the need for sleep during the night. With regular exercise during the day sleeplessness is usually not too bothersome. However, elderly patients who complain of changes in their sleeping habits are often reassured to know that the phenomenon is not uncommon among their contemporaries.

I was surprised by the minimal sleep requirements of Khfaf Lasuria, age about 130: "I go to bed at midnight and get up with the birds," she said. When she worked on the collective farm there was not time to nap, but in the last two years of retirement she finds little to do and naps regularly after the noon meal. In the winter she goes to bed earlier and sleeps later, but "I never needed much sleep; it is not my nature."

It is apparent that regular vigorous physical activity throughout life is an important factor promoting well being and longevity. The major benefit of exercise is to the heart and circulation. One is never too old to commence a regular program of exercise and, once started, will never grow too old to continue it.

7

GENETICS

Prescription for a long life: Choose your parents
carefully.

Anonymous

Long-lived individuals generally have long-lived parents or close relatives. This fact made me wonder whether genetic factors played a dominant role in the concentration of old people I saw in Vilcabamba and Hunza. Both contained small groups of individuals who had lived in extreme isolation for several centuries—in the case of Hunza perhaps 2000 years. It seemed that a genetic tendency to long life might account for the many old people in both communities. There is no gene for longevity, as far as we know. There are only "bad" genes which can increase the probability of contracting or developing a fatal illness. If the forebears of the present-day Vilcabambans or Hunzakuts lacked such "bad" genes it is possible, at least, that this lack might express itself as an unusual longevity in later inbred generations. This is possible, though the general expectation from close intermarriages among humans is actually a deterioration of the species. In fact, Alex Comfort has shown that offspring of genetically diverse members of a species are likely to be unusually vigorous and long-lived—so-called "hybrid vigor." Nevertheless, it is possible that inbreeding of humans who lacked bad genes might result in a cluster of long-lived individuals as seen in Vilcabamba and Hunza.

The situation in the Caucasus seemed to negate the primacy of genetic factors in the longevity seen there. In one relatively small area in Abkhasia on the Black Sea I saw centenarians derived from several different ethnic groups. Thus Russians, Georgians, Armenians, Georgian Jews, and Turks all contributed to the elderly population there. This strongly suggests the importance of local environmental factors. Nevertheless, when I interrogated each of the old people it became quickly apparent that they all had parents or brothers and sisters who also lived to very advanced ages. Thus genetic factors cannot be disregarded even in the Caucasus.

The importance of genetic factors in determining the life span becomes apparent when differences in longevity among species are compared. Rats very rarely exceed four years; cats, thirty years; horses, forty years; elephants, sixty years. The longest-lived species of mammal is man. There is considerable debate regarding whether some absolute biological limit to the human life span exists. (This will be considered in more detail later when the interesting results of tissue culture are described.) Even if such an absolute biological limit does exist, what ultimate age it permits is not known. That is why there is so much interest in documenting carefully the records of unusual human longevity since from such data may come an appreciation of the possible limits of the human life span. Most authorities have regarded claims of life span beyond 115 years to be unsubstantiated and spurious. I have taken the position that with documents of birth kept for only a minute fraction of the world's population one hundred years ago, one cannot afford to be dogmatic that all unusual claims are a priori false. We simply don't know enough today to afford a dogmatic position.

One puzzling feature regarding the incontestable genetic factor in determining longevity is its survival value to the species. From the information I could obtain from physicians in Russia, it seems that the old women of Georgia pass through their menopause in their mid-fifties rather than late forties to early fifties as do women in America. There may be a difference of five to eight years in the average age of women at menopause. This means, of course, that the extension of life span of these female centenarians is largely during their postreproductive period. Old males may retain their fertility to a much more advanced age, with sperm production persisting until close to 100 years. However, offspring by such elderly males, though alleged, must be exceedingly rare.

Generally only factors which increase fecundity and survival through the procreative life span are selectively retained in subsequent generations. How a feature, longevity, which expresses itself after the period of procreation is promoted by natural selection thus is not clear. From an evolutionary point of view, it is difficult to postulate genetic effects occurring after the reproductive period. It is this argument which leads to the conclusion previously expressed, that there is no "good" gene for longevity per se, only "bad" genes which may increase the likelihood of our developing some fatal illness. Perhaps the number of progeny of long-lived parents is actually greater than the average or that a higher degree of fecundity is also linked genetically to a factor or factors that promote long life—e.g. an enzyme that may enhance the disposal of cholesterol. Theodosius Dobzhansky has expressed this, stating, "We do not postulate specific genes which make life longer or shorter. It is a matter of genes acting during the entire life span of the organism, and being selected, for or against, according to the benefits or disadvantages they confer on the organism, with respect to its reproductive efficiency."

Several studies of life expectancy of children of long-lived parents indicate a significant advantage over offspring of short-lived parents. The advantage, however, is a modest one. In a detailed study of the inheritance of longevity based upon life insurance records, L. I. Dublin found that offspring of long-lived parents had a life expectancy at age twenty that probably does not exceed by three years the expectancy of a similar aged group whose parents were short-lived. This was the maximal statistical advantage that Dublin could attribute to heredity according to his examination of insurance records. Of course, even a three-year mean advantage in life span for offspring of long-lived parents might, in an individual instance, be compatible with an extension of life span long beyond this average figure. Such, in fact, must be the case when the lives of many offspring of long-lived parents will be shortened by accidental deaths which prevent the hereditary tendency for a long life from exhibiting itself.

One way to assess genetic versus environmental factors in determining longevity is through the examination of twins. There are two kinds of twins, monozygotic (one egg) and dizygotic (two-egg). Monozygotic or identical twins arise from a single fertilized egg. They have the same complement of genes and their heredity is identical. They, of course, must be both of the same sex. Differences between them must be the result of different environmental factors affecting each member of the pair. Dizygotic, or fraternal, twins by contrast each arise from separate ova fertilized by two different spermatozoa. They differ as much as two ordinary offspring of the same parents, who will have on the average fifty percent of their genes in common. Some will, therefore, resemble each other closely, while others will differ as strikingly as may two siblings.

A long-term study of twins aged sixty years and over was commenced by F. J. Kallman and has been continued by L. F. Jarvik to evaluate genetic influences on the life span. Comparison of monozygotic twin partners theoretically permits assessment of the effect of environmental variation on their identical genetic backgrounds. Comparison of dizygotic twins by contrast reflects the interaction of environmental and genetic factors. In a study of such twin pairs one expects to find fewer differences in identical twins than in fraternal twins. For instance, there will be similarities in diseases, types of illnesses and so forth in identical twins. There will also be many more differences in height, weight, body configurations in fraternal than in identical twins. It has been found by Kallman and associates that the differences between fraternal twins in ages reached at death also varied a great deal. As one would expect, there were greater differences in longevity between fraternal twins than identical twins. On the average monozygotic twins die within five years of each other though pairs have been observed in which differences in age at death exceeded a decade. The difference in age at death for dizygotic twins was much larger. This held true even for the oldest pairs despite the fact that the older a pair of twins become the greater is the likelihood of both members of the pair dying within a short time of each other. The male twins generally had shorter life spans than did female pairs. From such observations on twins it is concluded that genetic factors do affect longevity.

In all societies in which the risk of childbearing has been reduced so as to minimize the likelihood of maternal deaths, women outlive men. In the United States the 1970 census figures indicate a ratio of females to males at age seventy is three to two and at age ninety this ratio becomes two to one. Interestingly, there are slightly more baby boys born than baby girls according to the same census figures. The cross-over occurs at age eighteen, and from that age on females exceed males in an ever-increasing ratio. The explanation for this sex difference in longevity is not clear. A paper presented at the Gerontology Congress in Kiev in 1972 attributed the difference to an increased mortality among males because of the riskier, more hazardous existence which they live than that of the female. A more logically consistent explanation for the difference in longevity of the sexes I heard repeatedly in the Caucasus. Women, I was told, live longer than men because they are the stronger biologically. When I asked what the evidence was for this feminine biological superiority, I was told, women are biologically stronger than men because they live longer than men!

Although the difference in life span between male and female has been attributed to the more protected life of the human female, the difference most probably has a more fundamental basis. F. C. Madigan and R. B. Vance found a ten-percent female predominance in life expectancy of 9813 brothers and 32,041 sisters in American Catholic teaching orders. Thus even when male and female are presumably subjected to similar environmental stress situations the favorable life span differential for the female is present.

Jarvik points out that in every species in which sex-specific longevity variation has been studied the female outlives the male. For the fruitfly the differences range about ten percent (thirty-three versus thirty-one days)—and more than 2¹/₂ times for the spider (271 versus 100 days). From the point of view of the male not all of nature's arrangements in this regard smack of fair play. Consider the case of the praying mantis. Copulation in that species only occurs *after* the female bites off the head of the luckless male!

There has long been an interest in individual susceptibility to disease. Certain persons seem prone to develop certain diseases. Hippocrates, the father of medicine, was careful to distinguish between various types of patients. He attributed their differences to variations in the blend of "humors." Today we might refer to constitutional differences, still a vague but useful notion. The occurrences of many diseases in families points to a genetic basis for such constitutional differences. Among the illnesses that are major killers of our elderly, genetic factors play a significant but variable role and thus in a negative sense influence longevity.

Among the risk factors for heart attacks is paternal coronary heart disease. There is sufficient familial incidence of heart attacks to alert us to a definite genetic basis. But coronary heart disease is etiologically multifactorial, and only in the unusual circumstance can the means by which the genetic factor or factors causally effecting the occurrence of heart attacks be delineated. There have been studies indicating that differences in the caliber of the coronary arteries exist and the narrower vessels influence the incidence of heart attacks. Such differences in size of these critical blood vessels could have a genetic basis as well as be influenced by physical activity.

Elevation of blood lipid concentrations, especially of cholesterol and probably also of triglycerides (the major neutral fats), correlate with an increased incidence of coronary atherosclerosis. In some instances the high concentration of lipids in the blood can be shown to be genetically determined. For example in diabetes mellitus, which affects at least two million of our population, there is a strong hereditary basis and also an associated high incidence of vascular diseases, including coronary heart disease. Other forms of elevated blood lipids also follow a genetically determined pattern, but in most instances of coronary heart disease the possible role of genetic factors remains an area for speculation and the importance of dietary factors, physical activity, and other environmental factors are also receiving serious consideration.

The value of defining the genetic factors in the occurrence of heart disease would be to segregate a high-risk group who might benefit from an intensive application of prophylactic measures. Even where a genetic predisposition to develop coronary heart disease exists, it must be the interaction between this tendency and environmental factors to a greater or lesser degree that produces the final fatal outcome. Thus more research on both genetic and environmental factors is urgently needed, while such guides to the latter that have been discovered should be more widely applied to stop the ravages of the number one killer of adults in most of the Western countries.

The tendency for hypertension to cluster in families indicates a probable genetic basis for its occurrence. The distribution of hypertension in the population seems to follow a polygenic factor—i.e., several different genes contributing to its occurrence. In a few specific conditions, such as polycystic kidneys, a single-gene disturbance transmitted as a dominant defect is responsible. For the common form of hypertension, namely essential hypertension (the name expressing our ignorance of its cause or causes), there is no agreement on the contribution of hereditary versus environmental factors. Studies of twins indicate that genetic factors are operative in determining blood pressure, but they do not explain what the physiological basis for the elevated blood pressure may be nor the manner in which genetic factors may influence the several variables which can act to increase blood pressure. Hypertension is all too prevalent, having an incidence of one in five persons over the age of fifty-five. Since it is the major risk factor contributing to strokes as well as a probable factor in heart attacks it is a major deterrent to longevity today.

Next only to cardiovascular diseases, cancer is the major predator on our population aged sixty and above. The increasing incidence of cancer today is related to the extension of the human life span. Genetic factors play a very important role in some cancers and have a vaguely suggested significance in others. Cancer cells themselves generally exhibit a grossly abnormal chromosomal composition. Certain malignancies show specific chromosomal changes. The relationship between the so-called "Philadelphia chromosome" (chromosome 21 with a portion deleted) and the occurrence of leukemia is well established. Cancer affecting a specific organ such as breast or stomach is known to occur in higher incidence in the same organ among the relatives of the patient than in the general population. Experimental animals can be bred so that a high proportion of offspring develop spontaneous cancers.

All this evidence of genetic factors influencing the occurrence of cancer is complicated by the knowledge that viruses may be incorporated into the deoxyribonucleic acids of the genes—the material which carries the genetic information in our cells. Such transformed cells may have malignant properties. Thus genetic predisposition to a neoplasm may depend upon transmission of a viral infection from parent to offspring. However, viral infections which affect the genetic material of cells, predisposing them to cancer, may have effects not too different from the action of X rays or other radiant energy which may also cause chromosomal disorder that result in cancer. That X rays and viruses can induce cancer is unquestionable, but whether this effect resides in their ability to affect the genetic material of cells requires further investigation.

Interestingly, cancer cells are the only human cells which have escaped the constraints of aging and attained potential immortality. But this escape is associated with uncontrolled growth, which unfortunately terminates rather than liberates the host. As will be discussed later, understanding of the means by which transformed cells (cancer cells) have thrown off the constraints of a limited life span and thus attained immortality will undoubtedly contribute greatly to our understanding of the aging process. The relationship can hardly be fortuitous and will constitute a large advance when it is fully understood.

Genetic factors can influence the quality of life for the elderly as well as its duration by effects on the brain. There are some forms of presenile dementia—deterioration of the mind—which are clearly genetically linked. Alzheimer's disease, which may produce brain atrophy with a mental state similar to late stages of senile dementia but at age forty, is clearly hereditary. T. Larsson and coworkers in Stockholm demonstrated a fourfold greater risk of developing senile dementia among the relatives of patients with senile dementia than for the population in general. From his study of twins over age sixty and their relatives, Kallman concluded that several genetic factors played a role in the etiology of senile dementia. The risk of senile dementia was greatest for the co-twin of a pair of monozygotic twins when one of the pair was afflicted. However, the risk in the incidence of senile psychosis was significantly increased in two-egg twins and even among siblings. Our understanding of senile dementia is so rudimentary that conjecture regarding the means by which genetic factors affect the occurrence of senile dementia—the degenerate brain syndrome of old age—would be only idle speculation.

Recently a combination of techniques have been brought to bear on the nature of some of the hereditary or genetically determined factors we have been discussing. Epidemiologic studies have conclusively established the role of cigarette smoking in the occurrence of cancer of the lung. Still, differences in susceptibility among smokers to this dread consequence are great. One possible explanation for the marked differences in susceptibility has been reported. It has been shown that the tars from the cigarette smoke must first undergo a chemical change, *hydroxylation*, to become carcinogenic. The enzyme, aryl hydrocarbon hydroxylase, which is capable of catalyzing this hydroxylation, was found present in much greater quantities in smokers who developed lung cancer than in smokers who did not. Thus a genetic factor—the presence of the aryl hydrocarbon hydroxylase—is necessary in order that an exogenous or environmental cause of cancer, namely smoking, can have its noxious effect. Understanding of the details of carcinogenesis may be expected to yield screening procedures which will tell us who is at risk in the public at large and assist us in developing means of protecting such individuals.

The counterpart to the examination of coincidences or differences in the medical history of identical twins would be the study of two different populations exposed to an identical environment. This is a situation that is difficult to achieve in actuality because cultural practices may make environmental influences less "identical" than superficial appearances would lead one to expect. However, looking across the narrow expanse of the Hunza River from Hunza to the neighboring state of Nagir on the opposite bank I speculated on what an excellent control it would be for what I saw in Hunza. Although the Hunza River alone separates the two states, a perpetual animosity between the peoples of Hunza and Nagir prevented intermarriages. Only the royal families of the two states were linked by marriage. The present Rani of Hunza was from the ruling family of Nagir, and the present crown prince of Hunza had been betrothed to the daughter of the Mir of Nagir—until he broke tradition to marry a college sweetheart in Lahore. Major John Biddulph, after a visit in these parts in 1876, records in his *Tribes of the Hindoo-Koosh,* "between Hunza and Nagir a great rivalry, which frequently resulted in open hostility, has always existed. . . . The division of the country into a number of small isolated communities has placed great restrictions on free intermarriage. . . . " The lack of intermarriage between these two people living under very similar conditions would seem to provide an excellent opportunity to compare their health and longevity. Separated only by the river, environmental influences seem nearly identical, and any significant differences might safely be attributed to genetic differences. Unfortunately there were not the time or facilities for me to visit Nagir and conduct such studies. I was told repeatedly in Hunza that, though Nagir was endowed with more fertile lands and readily available water supplies, the people of Nagir were not so healthy, long-lived, industrious, prosperous, or even as honest as the Hunzakuts. In leaving Hunza I did obtain permission to travel by the jeep route on the Nagir side of the valley since the Hunza road was blocked by landslides. As we drove through Nagir we encountered only two old men both in their eighties, and they and others corroborated all that we had heard about the superiority of the Hunzakuts. Interestingly, the differences between the two peoples is explained in the native mind as due to the shorter hours of sunshine on the Nagir side because Nagir is in the shadow of Mt. Rakaposhi—a purely environmental rather than a genetic explanation!

SEX AND AGE

Moses was an hundred and twenty years old when he died: his eye was not dim, nor his natural force abated.

Deuteronomy, 34:7

An active interest in the opposite sex is regarded in the popular mind as the *sine qua non* of vigor and vitality. One is reminded of the lines of "It Ain't Necessarily So" from *Porgy and Bess:* "Methuselah lived 900 years—but who calls that livin' when no gal'll give in to no man what's 900 years?" In fact, the boastful nature of the male in most societies regarding his prowess in this realm makes it quite difficult to obtain reliable information about sexual activity in the elderly. Although the ovaries of women do stop functioning at the menopause, usually in the late forties or early fifties, this climacteric event has little influence on libido. Likewise, in the male aging is associated with a gradual decrease in the number of cells in certain organs, including the testes. The germinal cells which produce sperm are affected first, but later the cells which manufacture testosterone, the major male sex hormone, may also diminish in number and activity. Still, sexual potency in the male may persist to advanced old age. In the United States, Herman Brotman of the Department of Health, Education, and Welfare states that among the twenty million Americans over the age of sixty-five there are approximately 3500 marriages every year and that "sex as well as companionship are given as the reasons."

Miguel Carpio, age 110 and the oldest citizen of Vilcabamba, smokes and drinks, and his daughter says that he still likes to flirt with the girls. According to her, "He was quite a ladies' man in his younger days." Says he: "I can't see them too well anymore, but by feeling I can tell if they are women or not." Then he laughs, happy at the reaction from his audience. Yet Miguel Carpio was married only once. His wife died at the age of eighty-three, twenty-seven years ago. When asked if he would like to turn back the clock, Miguel Carpio thought for a long time and replied, "I would not wish to be fifteen again, but if I could take off fifteen years from my age that would be wonderful. . . .Fifteen years ago I was in better condition than I am now; my eyesight was fine and I felt good." He was nearly ninety-five then.

Dr. Salvador told us that most of the older males in Vilcabamba have continuing sexual activity and generally have had children by other women besides their wives. However, there has never been violence resulting from jealousies among the villagers over such relationships.

In the Caucasus we asked the old people to what age they thought youth extends. Gabriel Chapnian, age 117, of Gulrepsh, gave a typical response: "Youth normally extends up to the age of eighty, but with me I was still young then." The youngest age cited was sixty. Quado Jonashia, a neighbor, age 111 years, was moderately embarrassed at our question as we were accompanied by a woman doctor from the regional health center. He thought "youth" meant engaging in sexual activity and admitted that he considered himself a youth until "a dozen years ago." His formula for a long life is "No smoking, a lot of physical work, a good diet, and lots of drink." In answer to what he would like to do during the next fifty years, he said, "I'm going to marry if I can find a girl who suits me—at least I want to." He would like to relive his life and said, "If I started now with life much better, I think I would live 200 years rather than 100."

In Abkhasia it is customary for the men to marry late but for the bride to be quite young. Most men there married when thirty to forty years old. Chu Khasheeg of Hopee is 113 years old. He had been a shepherd and hunter but retired twelve years ago. He first married at the age of sixty and has five children: the oldest is forty-three and the youngest is thirty-two years old. He laughingly explained his late marriage: "I was too busy caring for my goats and sheep to think about women." Markhti Tarkhil, age 104 years, lives in the mountain village of Duripshi. He married when he was forty years old. "I still feel young. I sleep well, ride my horse, eat well, and swim every day, so I still feel like a youngster though I'm not as strong as I once was." When asked whether he still liked girls, Markhti rose and responded with true masculine bravado, "Come, I'll show you."

Nikolai Metravili, head of the collective farm at Duripshi, explained that there were two main reasons for late marriages among men. "Tradition dictates that you must wait until all your older brothers are married before taking a wife. Secondly, no one will trust you with his daughter until you have proven your worth both morally and economically and that takes until at least thirty to forty years of age." Although marriage is put off until forty, he claimed, there is no opportunity for premarital heterosexual activity. The villages are small, explained Metravili, everyone knows everyone else, and there are no loose women. Any encroachment on another's woman would draw swift and fatal reprisal. In most cases marriages had been arranged by relatives, as in Hunza, but love marriages are common now. The old people don't decry the current tendency toward early marriages. They acknowledge that conditions are different today, the young people are better educated, are economically independent at an earlier age, and are ready for the responsibilities of marriage.

Professor G. Z. Pitzkhelauri, a gerontologist in Soviet Russia, had collected some interesting figures relating marital status to longevity. Only married persons attain old age, he claims. In examining over 15,000 old persons, he found nearly all were or had been married. Many elderly couples had been married seventy, eighty, or even 100 years, and he thinks marriage and a regular prolonged sex life are very important to longevity. (But who can say which is cart and which is horse?) Women who had many children tend to live longer. His figures showed that among the centenarians only 2.5 percent of marriages were childless, whereas forty-four percent of the women had four to six children, twenty-three percent had only two to three children, nineteen percent had seven to nine children, and five percent had ten to fifteen offspring. Several women had even more than twenty children! Their offspring too were very fertile. Old men often remarry younger women when they are widowed, but old women generally do not remarry. Some old men have had three or four wives during their long life span.

It was noticeable that, while our society has adopted an increasing permissiveness of sexual expression among the young, in Abkhasia a greater freedom is granted to the elderly. In spite of this, overt expressions of affection in public are not deemed proper. Selac Butba, age 121, of Atara, kept laughing and joking throughout our interview: "Although you can't see through my clothes," he said, "be assured that underneath I have everything, all right!" He had nine children and added, "I'm an expert in producing children." However, when asked to sit closer to his wife for a photograph he responded, "Custom doesn't allow us to sit so close together in public—but, if you insist, I'll have to kiss her."

Until recently there has been very little factual information available regarding the scope of sexual behavior in the elderly. This has been a topic enshrouded by taboos which have inhibited both the elderly, on the one hand, from providing data, and physicians and behavioral scientists, on the other, from collecting information. The "dirty old man" view by our society of any expression of sexual interest by an elderly male understandably inhibits overt expression of such interests, even in the course of legitimate studies. Furthermore, even if cooperation of the elderly may be obtained for studies, relatives will become upset and are likely to intervene and obstruct participation. Respectable oldsters are thought not to have an interest in sex, and, if they do, it is believed that they should have the prudence to keep the interest to themselves.

Investigators themselves have inhibitions which prevent them from asking questions regarding sexual activity of the elderly. This reticence and embarrassment is not easily overcome. In the course of interviewing and examining villagers in Vilcabamba our young physician from Quito would ask each adult about his or her sexual activity. The young doctor turned to me with a look of distress and embarrassment as a 105-year-old spinster approached in line, and he asked me, "Do I have to ask her all those questions, too?" I found myself unable to insist that he must.

The cause of our inhibitions regarding sex in the elderly stems undoubtedly from several sources. Remnants of a Victorian prudishness are undoubtedly still with us, and even most physicians are uncomfortable in seeming to pry into the private lives of their patients. Dr. Eric Pfeiffer, a member of the Duke University Center for the Study of Aging and Human Development who has made important contributions from his studies on this subject, noted that, in a study of sexual behavior among the elderly in which he participated, young physician–investigators found it difficult to inquire into the sexual lives, past or present, of aged spinsters. There were fourteen such women voluntarily in his study group, but from only four of these had the interrogator obtained any data on sexual behavior.

Since sexual activity after the menopause cannot lead to procreation, it is not countenanced by those who believe sexual activity has no other function. However, even the permissiveness of our present culture, which recognizes a recreative as well as a procreative role for sex, does not extend to the elderly.

Pfeiffer points out that the taboo against sex in old age is, in part, an extension of the incest taboo. Children in our society often experience a great deal of anxiety from observing or imagining their parents engaged in sexual activity. Since the elderly represent the parent generation, some of the discomfort in considering sex activity among the elderly may be accounted for on this basis.

Not only does our society generally regard the elderly as asexual, but it has developed a series of cultural stereotypes which effectively restrain the elderly from expressing themselves on the subject. Thus, most people believe that sexual desire and sexual activity cease with the onset of old age, and that those elderly who claim to be sexually active are either morally perverse or boastful and deceptive. In the face of such public prejudgment who would care to speak up? Nevertheless, the data of Kinsey, of Masters and Johnson, and of the longitudinal studies of the Duke University Center for the Study of Aging and Human Development have begun to bring factual information to this subject. In the longitudinal study the same individuals were repeatedly interviewed over a number of years so that changes in attitudes and behavior with time could be determined in the same individual.

Kinsey included only a very meager sample of elders in his extensive study of male sexuality. Of the 12,214 men in his study, there were only 106 men over the age of sixty, only eighteen of whom were over the age of seventy. Thus, his conclusions about elderly men are based on small numbers. Nevertheless, he arrived at some conclusions which he felt his data justified. With male sexuality, aging begins at adolescence. Sexual activity in the male is greatest during late adolescence (ages sixteen through twenty) and ability then diminishes; there is no point at which old age suddenly enters the picture. The rate at which males slow up at ages above sixty does not exceed the rate at which they had been slowing up and ceasing activity in the previous age groups. Starting from a high point of 3.2 orgasms per week for the single males, or 4.8 for the married males, in the middle teens, the mean for the unmarried and married who engage in sexual activity drops steadily to about the same point: 1.8 per week at fifty years, to 1.3 per week at sixty years, and 0.9 per week at seventy years of age. His figures show no sudden decrease in sexual activity to support the popular notion of a male climacteric occurring in middle age, with its postulated sudden loss of sexual interest and activity. However, he also found that there was a rapid rise in the proportion of elderly study subjects who were impotent. His figures showed a rise from eighteen percent at age sixty to twenty-seven percent at age seventy.

As to the causes of this gradual sexual decline with age, he regarded psychologic fatigue or monotony as an undoubted factor. How much of the overall decline in the rate for the older male is physiologic, how much is based on psychologic situations, how much is based on the reduced availability of contacts, and how much is dependent upon preoccupation with other social or business functions in the professionally most active period of the male's life it was impossible for him to state. He also noted that married men, compared with single men or with men who had previously been married, had frequencies of sexual activity which were only slightly higher than those of their unmarried counterparts. It would seem, therefore, that being elderly and single carries with it no sexual disadvantage for the male over being elderly and married.

Kinsey's sample of elderly females was also small, including only fifty-six over the age of sixty out of a total number of 5940 women studied. The mean frequency of orgasm for the total sample rises gradually at ages twenty-six to thirty and falls gradually with age thereafter. However, the decline in frequency of orgasm, he believes, reflects the declining activity of the male partner, and he states that there is little evidence of aging in the sexual capacities of the female until late in her life. In contrast to men, however, the single or previously married female had rates of sexual activity markedly below that of her married peers.

Masters and Johnson devote a considerable portion of their book *Human Sexual Response* to the aging male and female. There is no question, they state, that the human male's sexual responsiveness wanes as he ages. This is true if sexual responsiveness is judged by (1) existing levels of sexual excitement, (2) ability to make coital connection, (3) ability to terminate coition with ejaculation, and (4) the incidence of masturbation or of nocturnal emissions, as well as of coitus. In their observations of 212 male subjects whose ages ranged from fifty-one to ninety years, they found a major difference exists between the response pattern of males age forty-one to sixty years and of those past the age of sixty. This difference is a loss of maintained levels of sexual expression. But the aging male's sexual capacity and performance varies from individual to individual and from time to time in a particular individual.

The most important factor in the maintenance of effective sexuality for the aging male is a continued and regular sexual performance. A male who has sustained a high level of sexual activity during his early adulthood and who is repeatedly and regularly stimulated during middle age is likely to sustain sexual activity into old age if given the opportunity. They found that, although secondary impotence (inability to attain an erection for psychological reasons) increases markedly after the age of fifty years, the male over fifty years old can be trained out of his secondarily acquired impotence in a high percentage of cases.

Masters and Johnson also state that the male over the age of fifty whose sexual activity may have been dormant for physical or social reasons may be restimulated if the male wishes to return to active sexual practices and has a cooperative partner. If he is in adequate health, little is needed to support adequacy of sexual performance in a seventy- or even eighty-year-old male other than some available partner and psychologic reason for reactivated sexual interest.

Obviously, sexual capacity and performance are influenced by acute or chronic physical infirmity or by the general physiologic involution of the total body. However, Masters and Johnson found that the waning sexual activity of the elderly male could usually be classified as due to one of the following reasons: (1) monotony of a repetitious sexual relationship (usually expressed as boredom with a partner); (2) preoccupation with career or economic pursuits; (3) mental or physical fatigue; (4) overindulgence in food or drink; (5) physical infirmities of either the individual or his spouse; (6) fear of inability to perform with the partner leading to avoidance of activity rather than possible humiliation from impotence.

Loss of interest due to monotony in a sexual relationship is probably the most common cause of decreased sexual activity in the aging male, they claim. An activity which depends on the arousal of a high state of excitement in the male doesn't flourish on a routinized performance. The female partner who elicits boredom may herself be distracted by demands of children, social activities, her own career, or any number of personal interests outside of her marriage. Masters and Johnson state that many of the women they interviewed by their own admission no longer showed either sexual interest in, or sexual concern for, their husbands. In addition to a loss of interest in sex, the aging female partner may be thought to lose physical attractiveness and therefore cease to be sexually stimulating.

Physical infirmity of the aging female partner is an ever-increasing factor in limiting the aging male in his sexual opportunities. With loss of sexual outlet many aging males will report rapid loss of sexual tension. The situation of an aging husband with a physically infirm wife may not be as restrictive as is the case of the aging wife with a physically infirm husband. In our culture the aging male has much more opportunity for sexual outlet than does the aging female.

With aging in the male, Masters and Johnson noted a qualitative as well as quantitative change. All stages of sexual arousal, excitement as well as orgasm, are more sluggish and less intense than in the younger male. The older male takes longer to arrive at a full penile erection, but once achieved erection may be maintained for extended periods of time without ejaculation even when the variety and effectiveness of sexual stimulation is sustained. The vasocongestion and muscle tensions which accompany the sexual act are diminished in the aging male.

Nevertheless, Masters and Johnson concluded that, if elevated levels of sexual activity are maintained from early years and neither acute nor chronic physical incapacity intervenes, aging males usually are able to continue some form of active sexual expressions into the seventy- or even eighty-year age groups. Even if coital activity has been avoided for long periods of time, men in these age groups can be returned to effective sexual function if adequate stimulation is instituted and interested partners are available.

In the aging female there is also a qualitative change in the sexual response. The reaction of non-genital tissues of the body, as well as the changes in the genitals resulting from vasocongestion and muscle tensions during sexual excitement are diminished in the aging woman as compared with the young woman. In the postmenopausal state the lack of the ovarian hormone, estrogen, results in involution of the target organs, i.e., the labia, vagina, uterus, breasts. Instead of the corrugated, thick, reddish mucosa of the vaginal wall of a young woman, there is a thinning and pallor of the mucosa and a shortening of both the vaginal length and width in the estrogen-lacking postmenopausal female. Vaginal lubrication, which is a very prompt reaction to sexual arousal in the young woman, is delayed in the aging female. Orgasm is likely to be less intense and less sustained in the aging female.

How much of the diminished reaction is due to estrogen lack is still not clear. Certainly discomfort during coitus which results from insufficient lubrication, uterine cramping, and thinning of the vaginal wall as well as atrophy and loss of elasticity may result from lack of hormone. But sexual interest and responsiveness seems to be largely independent of estrogen. With opportunity for regular intercourse, the elderly female will retain a far higher capacity for sexual performance than her female counterpart who does not have similar opportunities. Hormonal lack thus has only an indirect influence upon, but certainly not absolute control over, female sexual capacity or performance.

For many women, Masters and Johnson observed, the menopause is the occasion for a renewed sexual interest and activity. The assurance against the possibility of pregnancy that the menopause affords is one of the most frequently occurring factors responsible for increased sexual feelings evident in women in the fifty-to-sixty-year-old age group.

The data of Masters and Johnson confirm the earlier conclusion of the Kinsey group that a large part of the sex drive during the postmenopausal age is directly related to the sexual habits established during the procreative years. A woman who had a happy, well-adjusted, and stimulating marriage may progress through the menopausal and postmenopausal years with little or no interruption in the frequency of, or interest in, sexual activity.

On the other hand, for women who have been unable to establish regularly recurrent psychologically satisfactory sexual relations at an earlier age, the menopause is likely to be associated with a decrease in sex drive. For those women who have regarded sex as repugnant, the menopause may serve as an excuse to cease all further sexual activity.

The woman above the age of sixty is very dependent upon male adequacy. When available the male marital partner is on the average four years older than the female partner. Many of the older husbands are suffering from some physical disability or senescence which makes sexual activity with them unattractive or impossible. Thus it is often the case that the elderly married woman who might still be interested in continued heterosexual activity may be denied this opportunity because of physical infirmity of her mate. Needless to say, extramarital sexual partners are not likely to be available to women in this age group. The diminished frequency of sexual outlet of the elderly female is more a reflection of the decreasing adequacy of her male partner than of decrease in her capabilities or, often, of her interest.

The trend toward increasing longevity in our society with the longer life span for the female than for the male must, of necessity, deprive many aging females the opportunity for heterosexual relations. Masturbation may be the substitute for the elderly female lacking a male partner. Women who never marry and who have employed this technique during their twenties and thirties usually continue the same pattern for relief of sexual tensions into their sixties.

The two concluding paragraphs of Masters and Johnson's chapter on the aging female summarize their investigations and thoughts. "There seems to be no physiologic reason why the frequency of sexual expression found satisfactory for the younger woman should not carry over into the postmenopausal years. The frequency of sexual intercourse or manipulative activity during the postmenopausal years is of little import, as long as the individuals are healthy, active, well-adjusted members of society.

"It would seem that the maladjustments and abnormalities of sex drive shown by hyper- or hyposexuality [increased or decreased sexual interest and activity] which develop during and after the menopause might best be treated by prophylaxis. If satisfactory counseling of sexual content were made more available to sexually insecure, uneducated or inadequate women in the premenopausal years, there is reason to believe that the unresolved tensions of the later years might be reduced or, to a large extent, avoided. There is no reason why the milestone of the menopause should be expected to blunt the human female's sexual capacity, performance, or drive. The healthy aging woman normally has sex drives that demand resolution. The depths of her sexual capacity and the effectiveness of her sexual performance, as well as her personal eroticism, are influenced indirectly by all of the psycho- and sociophysiologic problems of her aging process. In short, there is no time limit drawn by the advancing years to female sexuality."

The Duke longitudinal study also found that sexual interest and coital activity are by no means rare in persons beyond age sixty. However, their findings differ somewhat from the impression one has from reading Masters and Johnson's report. It was found, in the 254 subjects ranging initially from sixty to ninety-four years of age in the Duke study, that about eighty percent of the men whose health, intellectual status, and social functioning were not significantly impaired reported continuous sexual interest at the start of the study, and this proportion did not decline significantly ten years later. However, in this same group of men, seventy percent were sexually active at the start of the study, whereas ten years later this proportion had dropped to twenty-five percent. Thus there is a gross discrepancy between the number still interested in sex and the number still engaging in sexual activity.

Among the women whose health, intellectual status, and social functioning were satisfactory, only about one-third reported continuing sexual interest, and this proportion did not change significantly over a ten-year period of observation. However, only about one-fifth of the same group of healthy elderly females reported at the start of the study that they were engaging in regular sexual activity. This proportion did not decline during the ten years of observation. Thus, far fewer elderly women than men were still interested in sex or sexually active.

It is encouraging that such studies are revealing factual information about sexual interests and activity among the elderly. The picture that emerges is quite different from the bland asexual image most have of the elderly. The facts, which are still meager and quite inadequate, should afford some reassurance to many who look with fear upon their impending old age. Certainly for many it must be the thought of losing sexual interest and capability with advancing years which makes the future look gloomiest. It is apparent that for the healthy, well-adjusted, socially functional person who has enjoyed regular sexual activity, the capability—physiologically at least—for such continued enjoyment exists well into advanced years.

Sexual activity is, of course, not a requirement for a long life. But since sex is one of the gifts nature has provided to add enjoyment, zest and fulfillment to our existence, it plays a significant role in our lives. Since my thesis is that the well-adjusted, happy, confident, and socially productive person is one likely to live long, in this context, a continuing and healthy sexual adjustment is important throughout the total life span.

The importance of a happy marriage to longevity was emphasized by a 100-year-old Azerbaijanian who had married his seventh wife only three years previously. "My first six wives were all wonderful women," he reported, "but this present wife is an angry woman, and I have aged at least ten years since I married her. If a man has a good and kind wife, he can easily live 100 years."

THE BRAIN
AND AGING

The true way to render age vigorous is to prolong the youth of the mind.

Mortimer Collins (1827–1876) *The Village Comedy*, Part I

Picasso worked long hours on his paintings until age ninety-one. Verdi composed *Falstaff* at age eighty and his *Four Sacred Pieces* at eighty-five. Goethe completed his epic *Faust* at eighty-two. Churchill led the English as their prime minister at age eighty-one. Dr. Paul Dudley White at eighty-five was one of the first Westerners to visit Red China in 1971. When I arrived in Sukhumi I had a list of centenarians to visit there. We called at the home of Ichabod Shomerashvili, age 109, a Georgian Jew and were told by relatives that the old man had just left the past year and emigrated to Israel—a prime age to start a new life!

We have all known very elderly persons who were keen and sharp mentally, whose conversations were sprightly, and whose remarks and thoughts were well worth heeding. Others have become bumbling caricatures of their former selves. It is this preservation of mental function that is so essential to the quality of life we seek in old age, and senility is what we all fear.

It is possible to speak with more assurance regarding the structural anatomic changes which occur in the brain with time than of the accompanying functional alterations. It is a general biological principle that the less specialized a cell remains the more readily can it replenish itself. The cells which make up our central nervous system are among the most highly differentiated and specialized of cells. In so becoming they have paid the price in an inability of the mature nerve cell to divide and replicate. If liver tissue is removed surgically, the remaining cells promptly multiply and largely replace what has been removed. Not so with the brain; any nerve cell that dies is a permanent loss. Sacrificing the ability to regenerate apparently is essential for the stable information storage and communications functions of the brain. These functions reside in the complex network of synapses (cell-to-cell contacts). The integration of the nervous system acquired through synapses is central to the cortical functions, such as intelligence. The number of cells in the brain is established during the late embryonic period and the first year or so of postnatal life. This is why development of the brain is so vulnerable during these early formative stages to noxious influences both internal and external. In later life brain cells can be damaged or destroyed, but no new ones can be created.

Since all nonreplicating cells must have a finite life span—and this applies to brain cells—depopulation will occur with aging. It has been estimated that the human central nervous system contains some twenty billion nerve cells, and this number gradually dwindles after age thirty at a constant rate. Atrophy and weight loss of the brain are the most common features of aging of the nervous system. One estimate is that the loss amounts to some one-third of the cell content at age 100 and that the decline occurs at a uniform rate with age. The maximal weight of the brain reflecting its cell content occurs between ages twenty and thirty, and the subsequent decrease in weight is about seventeen percent by eighty years of age. This progressive atrophy of the brain corresponds to a numerical loss of neurons (nerve cells) and their associated processes and supporting cells. It is known that there exists no direct correlation between intelligence of an individual and the weight of his brain. Anatole France was found to have an unusually small brain, while some idiots have been found to have much larger brains. Whether a decrement in brain weight in a given individual must be associated with a loss of intellectual capacity is another matter—probably true if due to a loss of nerve cells in the cortex.

Neuropathologists have come to recognize certain microscopic changes which characterize the aging brain. The main changes include the accumulation of neuritic or senile plaques, accumulation of lipofuscin within nerve cells, and neurofibrillary tangles. The so-called senile plaques are already present in the brains of a small percent of persons in their thirties, and by age seventy ninety percent have them. With senile dementia their numbers increase and the size of individual plaques increases. They are not related to atherosclerotic disease in the blood vessels of the brain, and their relation to senile dementia is obscure in spite of their name. However, they are clearly an indication of damage to the affected nerve cells.

Of particular interest is the presence of a proteinaceous substance called amyloid within these microscopic plaques. This mysterious substance has been discovered in a variety of conditions and may deposit in any organ. When it accumulates in sizable amounts it generally interferes with normal tissue or organ function. Very recent studies have revealed that some amyloid is protein, and is part of the complex antibody molecule which "recognizes" foreign molecules (antigens) that appear in the body. The accumulation of amyloid supports a current theory which proposes that the aging process results from a mistake in identity whereby the immune system makes antibodies to normal body proteins rather than only to specific foreign proteins and thus destroys normal cells. The finding of deposits of portions of antibody molecules within these plaques may have relevance to this theory of aging. It remains to be proven, however, that the amyloid in brain is of this specific type.

The accumulation of the fatty pigment lipofuscin is the most universal age-related change within cells. Its presence is recognized in the heart, liver, and other organs as well as within the nervous system. Lipofuscin increases with time and appears as microscopic granules. The lipofuscin consists primarily of oxidized, unsaturated fats. Interestingly, the process is the same as that involved in the "drying" or hardening of oil-based paints. It is the uptake of atmospheric oxygen by the unsaturated vegetable oils in these paints which partially oxidizes and rigidifies the fats, producing the insoluble familiar tough coat. Within nerve cells these partially oxidized fats also are resistant to removal. Once formed within the cell they resist attack by the cell's "clean-up squad," the packets of enzymes which dissolve or digest unwanted intruders and prevent their accumulation within cells. The failure to digest this material allows it to accumulate with time. Generally its presence in small amounts within cells is thought not to adversely affect the function of the cell. However, when large amounts of lipofuscin crowd the cell interior the nerve cell may atrophy and lose its function.

Since lipofuscin consists of partially oxidized fats its accumulation may be expected to depend on the presence of unsaturated fats and of antioxidants. Unsaturated fats are found in vegetable and fish oils. As discussed earlier, they may have prophylactic value in preventing the development of atherosclerosis. It would be ironical if a diet high in unsaturated fats would protect the heart from atherosclerosis only to impair the brain with deposits of lipofuscin. Fortunately this dilemma is avoided if the diet also contains antioxidants.

Antioxidants are commonly encountered in our everyday experience. They are added to the antifreeze in our automobile radiators to prevent rusting (oxidation) of the iron of which the radiator is constructed. In our bodies vitamin E is the most important of the naturally occurring antioxidants. It is pertinent that experimental vitamin E deficiency in animals is associated with increased deposits of lipofuscin in cells. A major natural source of vitamin E in the diet is in grains. But as the latter are highly milled and refined their vitamin E content is diminished. Whole grains and wheat germ are especially rich sources of vitamin E. A therapeutic role for vitamin E in man has not been established and a clinical trial to determine its efficacy in preventing the accumulation of lipofuscin would be most difficult to evaluate. In a well-balanced, unrestricted diet no supplementation with this vitamin should be necessary, as is true for the other known vitamins as well.

Other microscopic changes in the brain also occur with aging but, as with the senile plaques and lipofuscin, these changes generally may also be found in normal brains from young individuals. Only the incidence of these changes increases with age, and their presence at any age is quantitatively increased in the presence of dementia. Dementia is the deterioration of intellectual faculties with associated emotional disturbances which result from organic brain disease. Senile dementia refers to the progressive deterioration of mental faculties and emotional stability which occur in some with old age.

The so-called Alzheimer's neurofibrillary tangles are, by contrast, not present in the cortex of brains (the outer layers of the hemispheres of the brain essential for intellectual activity) of normal persons. Normal nerve cells contain many fine fibrillar processes which make contact with neighboring nerve cells. Instead of the normal orderly display of these processes, the Alzheimer's neurofibrillary tangles are chaotic clumps of fibrils, like tangles of sewing thread. These tangles occur in high incidence in the cortex of the unfortunate elderly with senile dementia.

Until recently it was customary to attribute senile dementia to a reduced blood supply to the brain because of narrowing of the large arteries to the head from atherosclerosis. Now it is recognized that atherosclerotic changes are responsible for dementia in only a minority of cases among the elderly, whereas senile plaques and neurofibrillary tangles are responsible for senile dementia in the majority of instances. Not only is the loss of many brain cells involved, but structural abnormalities affecting a large fraction of the remaining cells must be present before senile dementia occurs. Atherosclerotic changes, which lead to small strokes with loss of brain substance, can be largely avoided by prevention or treatment of high blood pressure. We have, however, almost no understanding of factors that promote formation of senile plaques, neurofibrillar tangles, lipofuscin deposition, or degeneration of nerve cells. However, aging of the brain cannot be too different from aging in other organs; lipofuscin and amyloid accumulate in the heart and other organs as well with advanced age.

Changes in metabolism and function accompany the changes in structure. The decline in the metabolic rate of brain and of cerebral blood flow usually observed in aging patients is believed to be due principally to pathological conditions rather than to chronological age per se. Investigators have shown that in old persons who are in excellent health and have no apparent mental deterioration, the oxygen consumption and blood flow of the brain do not differ much from those of healthy young adults. On the other hand, it has been repeatedly observed that a reduction of cerebral oxygen consumption and cerebral blood flow is associated with an impairment in intellectual function. The major change in the brain wave (the electrical activity of the brain) of senescent subjects is a progressive slowing of the brain-wave rhythm.

There are functional accompaniments of these structural and physiologic changes in the brain with age. Certain declines and losses in mental capability are inevitable. All old people experience some decline in physical vigor and stamina; there is also a gradual decline in mental agility. Both motor and verbal responses are slowed. But responses to basic drives, such as hunger, are also less in older experimental animals. It has proven to be a most difficult problem in psychology to pinpoint the basis for the slowed responses by the elderly to a variety of different test situations. There seems to be a hint of indifference on the part of the elderly to attainment of high performance ratings in such test situations. Thus the factor of motivation may color the results of such psychological studies.

There can be little question that the elderly individual has difficulty in adapting to new situations. We all conserve mental effort by routinizing responses. When environmental conditions remain constant routine responses to a particular set of circumstances serve the individual well. But, when the conditions change and response patterns must be unlearned and new behavior acquired, the elderly fail in comparison with the young. Perhaps the best definition of aging is the gradual loss of adaptive ability with age. This definition embraces a loss of physiological adaptability, but also of mental adjustment with aging. Since the brain is the organ *par excellence* for adaptation by the human species, this loss with aging manifests itself in intellectual conservatism and in difficulty unlearning fixed response patterns and acquiring new responses that are effective and compatible with survival in our ever-changing world. It is the rapid rate of change in our world that puts a premium on the ability to acquire new responses; in a stable, traditional society the elderly may more readily remain adapted.

On the average, older persons do show changes, at least in degree, from the level of adaptive abilities shown by young healthy adults in the age range of twenty to thirty-nine years. R. M. Reitan has studied the psychologic changes associated with aging. He notes that the kinds of changes cited in the literature have included sensory limitations and slowness in response; a decline in intellectual efficiency especially in the area of abstraction ability; loss in the ability to comprehend conceptual problems; memory impairment, particularly relating to recent events; confusion in dealing with complex problems for which past experience is not immediately relevant; some tendency, particularly in unfamiliar surroundings, toward disorientation in time and place; reduction of activities and interests which may reach the point of apathy and emotional depression; impaired affect and diminished involvement with the environment; and rigidity or increased resistance to change.

The results of psychological tests by H. B. C. Reed and Ralph M. Reitan compared a young group with a mean age of twenty-eight years with an older group having a mean age of fifty-three years. The younger subjects were clearly superior to the older subjects on tests judged to be most dependent upon immediate adaptive ability. The older subjects were, however, slightly superior to the younger subjects on tests judged to be dependent upon memory and experience. The older subjects were markedly inferior to the younger subjects on tests of complex problem-solving procedures judged to be dependent upon immediate adaptive ability, whereas they were clearly not inferior on tests requiring stored information and experience. This type of finding has been confirmed.

Such specific deficits would seem to account for some of the changes with age mentioned earlier. These include loss in ability in abstraction and in the comprehension of complex problems, disorientation in time and space, and even recent-memory impairment. Deficits of these types could in time account for various reactions, such as reduction of activities and interests as well as rigidity and increased resistance to change.

Since the anatomical changes in the brain which were described result from a loss of functioning neurons, it is not surprising that older subjects show the same pattern of response on psychological testing that younger subjects with brain damage exhibit. Furthermore, since the brain is not independent of the health of other vital organs, Reitan has observed that tests in young subjects with relatively long-standing heart and lung disorders showed similarities with the results in subjects with brain damage and the nature of the psychologic deficits appear quite similar to the changes observed in older subjects. This constitutes confirmation of the old adage that a healthy mind can only exist in a healthy body.

The degree of social interaction generally decreases with advancing age. The deficiencies of older persons in dealing with situations requiring immediate problem-solving would lead them to limit their exploratory activities and result in an entrenchment and preoccupation with the familiar types of activities which past experience had taught could be dealt with competently. Thus, impairment of certain basic abilities in the elderly would predispose behavior toward conservatism, withdrawal, and disengagement.

Mental deterioration does not occur as an unrelated event in the aged. It is perhaps the best yardstick with which to measure physical deterioration as well. There is an association between psychological performance as measured with a battery of "intelligence tests" and longevity. In a group of twins initially sixty years or older, followed by Kallman and by Jarvik, psychological tests were done over a span of twenty years. The relationship between survival and psychomotor score was tested by comparing mean scores of the 168 twin subjects alive in 1955, the survivors, with those of the 100 twins whose demise antedated that year. The survivors had the higher mean scores at the time of the original testing.

Since the subjects were first tested at ages of sixty years or older, the higher mean scores of the survivors could be taken to reflect a relation between survival and initial level of ability rather than senescent decline. It was the rate of decline in performance, however, rather than the initial score that was associated with survival; slower decline was indicative of longer survival. Thus on retesting there was found to be a correlation between performance on certain psychological tests and survival; an increase in vocabulary score was more often associated with five-year survival than with death, while the reverse held true for a decrease in score.

Another aspect of the social problem of aging was succinctly expressed by one of my colleagues, who remarked, "You know, there really is no such thing as mental deterioration with aging; there are only distractions." As I have observed, many brilliant individuals lose scholarly productivity as their lives have become encumbered with a multitude of responsibilities which encroach upon time for reflection and independent thinking.

Although some of the age-related anatomical changes in the nervous system must be inevitable, there is no reason to believe that for most of us a healthy mental state cannot be preserved well into old age. The prerequisites are a healthy body and a positive frame of mind toward the world about us. When C. Judson Herrick stated, "You don't grow old; when you cease to grow, you are old," he was not referring to body growth, which is generally accomplished by age twenty, but to the development of continued interests and expanding mental horizons. The individuals mentioned in the introductory paragraph of this chapter all sustained broad interests in people and events about them and continued to learn and improve their understanding throughout their long lives. The untoward effects of physical inactivity and indolence on the body are easily recognized. It seems to be that mental laziness and torpor may have equally deleterious—if less visible—effects upon our intellects. Thus it should be possible by appropriate exercises to retain mental as well as physical activity.

10

PSYCHOLOGICAL AND SOCIAL FACTORS

All would live long, but none would be old.

Proverbs

A striking feature common to all three cultures was the high social status of the aged. Each of the very elderly persons we saw lived with family and close relatives—often an extended household—and occupied a central and privileged position within this group.

The sense of continuity of the family is strong. Khedzhgva Sukhba, age 105, of Hopee in Abkhasia, finds satisfaction and meaning in the continuity of her family. Thus, though her son left his wife pregnant when he went off to the army and failed to return, the wife gave birth to a son. This grandson also married and, recently, his wife produced a son. This continuity of sons, she said, gives her the greatest happiness.

Even those well over 100 for the most part continued to perform duties which were essential and contributed to the economy of the community in which they lived. A few hours of weeding in the fields, feeding the poultry, tending flocks, picking tea, washing the laundry, cleaning house, or caring for grandchildren performed on a regular daily basis continued to provide a sense of usefulness for the elderly. The agrarian societies to which these old people belong lend themselves to this kind of participation. In addition, the old people are esteemed for the wisdom that is thought to derive from long experience and their word in the family group is generally the law.

In Hunza this last point was evident in the mechanism by which the state is governed. Thus, the Mir holds court daily at 10 A.M. with his council of elders. The latter is comprised of some twenty wise old men from each of the villages in the kingdom. They sit in a circle on carpets spread at the foot of the Mir's wooden throne and listen to all disputes among the citizens and other domestic affairs. After a lively discussion (often including three or four elders talking simultaneously) with the Mir presiding and listening or talking too, a consensus is reached and the Mir announces his government's decision. Membership on the council of elders did not exempt the elders from work at home and obligations to their own family groups.

We had the good fortune to be in Hunza on the occasion of the wedding of the crown prince and thus to observe the traditional festive customs and costumes of the people. The celebrations with feasting and dancing went on for at least a week. Invariably it was the oldest man of each village who led the dance, and we recognized our acquaintances from the council of elders in this role. Occasionally a dance was enlivened by a sequence of hopping on one foot and then the other, but this was generally short lived. Such performances would continue for many hours while representatives from each village, complete in native costumes, had an opportunity to perform their dance and show their respect and allegiance. Women do not participate in these social activities and even in the audience they kept to sheltered positions, peering out from among trees or from rooftops behind the men.

We watched the strenuous, intricate performance of the folk dancers of Abkhasia in Sukhumi one evening with fascination. Interestingly, one dancer was dressed as a village elder and led and directed the dance group—symbolic recognition of the important role of the elderly in that society too. But their importance receives more than token recognition. Most continue with their work until the age of 100. There is no fixed or forced retirement age, and the elderly are not dismissed when they reach a certain age as occurs in our industrialized societies. Khfaf Lasuria of Kutol, age approximately 130, had applied for and received her old-age pension for only the past two years. Even when over 100 she was the recognized champion tea picker on her collective farm. When asked if he were helping in the construction of a new house springing up next to his, Selac Butba, age 121, responded, "Of course—they can't do without me." Temur Tarba, a vigorous, horse-riding member of the collective farm at Duripshi who had celebrated his hundredth birthday just three weeks before our visit, showed from his bearing and happy manner that he "had arrived." Only seven years earlier he had been designated as a Hero of Labor and was awarded this highest Soviet honor for his cultivation of corn. His father died at 110, his mother at 104, and an older brother died this year at 109. He smoked a good deal when we visited him, but he didn't inhale. He devotes the mornings to collecting tea and cultivating his garden. "It is best to be a youth," Temur states, "but I have good health, feel well, have wonderful children and I enjoy myself greatly now." Then he paused a moment and added, "Being one hundred is very special as each day is a gift."

We felt great sympathy for the ninety-eight- and ninety-nine-year-olds who were still nobodies in the presence of the centenarians. Of the 15,000 elderly persons over the age of eighty whom Professor Pitzkhelauri had studied, over seventy percent continue to be very active and more than sixty percent were still working on state or collective farms. They die quickly once a useful role in the community ceases.

People who no longer have a necessary role to play in the social and economic life of their society generally deteriorate rapidly. The pattern of increasingly early retirement in our own society takes a heavy toll of our older citizens. Industrialization caused a great migration from our farms to our cities in response to the needs for a labor force by factories and businesses. Mechanization of farming did much to maintain and increase productivity of farming so that fewer hands have been required. This too freed farm laborers of toil so that they moved to the cities, seeking jobs in our growing industries. But with automation of industry the need for laborers—except during times of rapid expansion, to keep our factories productive—has fallen off. The result has been a progressively earlier age of retirement and a shortening of the work week.

The retired person in our society all too often finds himself with no sustaining interests, with children who have no use for Dad or Mom, nor any room in their cramped urban apartments for parents. Even with economic independence the elderly find their children have moved away and made other friends and attachments. When visiting their children, they find their presence all too often tolerated rather than desired, especially if their visit becomes an extended one. They sense quickly that they have become a burden on their children, confirming in their own minds their uselessness. A search for friendship and companionship often drives them to centers where other retired elderly have congregated. The trailer parks in California, the hotels in Miami, and the housing and clubs for the elderly in every city are familiar examples of the retreat of the unneeded and often unwanted elderly from loneliness. All too often such groupings fail to satisfy the need.

One manifestation of this isolation and loneliness of our elderly is their high suicide rate. In 1966 the suicide rate was 10.9 persons per 100,000, but among aged white males the rate was four to six times higher than this average, and the incidence increases with age: 32.8 at ages fifty to fifty-four, 59.0 at ages above eighty-five. With the total number of suicides at 21,281 persons in 1966, 5,967 or twenty-eight percent were persons over the age of sixty.

Interestingly, the increasing suicide rate with age applies only to white males; the incidence is lower and declines with advanced age for our white female populations. Among nonwhite males and females the rate is lower and does not increase with age, though nonwhite males show a sudden increase in rate among those over eighty-five, and this is sevenfold greater than among nonwhite females in the same age grouping. The traditional female role as mother and housewife may protect her from the abrupt loss of role identity which suddenly confronts most males on retirement at age sixty-five to seventy. In fact, a sharp rise in suicide rate occurs over age seventy for white males.

These figures are undoubtedly minimal figures. Suicide is not sanctioned in our culture, and therefore reporting rates are prone to be falsely low. Diagnoses on death certificates from which these statistics are obtained often use the terms "accidental death" or "death by asphyxiation" to camouflage suicide by gunshot wounds or by carbon monoxide poisoning.

As one might expect, suicide rates are influenced by specific social situations in the lives of the elderly. The highest rates are among men who are divorced, followed by the widowed, and then by the unmarried. Suicide rates are lowest among persons with intact marriages. Other factors influencing suicide rates in the elderly are lack of employment, solitary living arrangements, and residence in deteriorating neighborhoods.

As continued technological advances accelerate the rate of change in our economy, the emphasis is on youth. In a traditional society like Hunza, which has changed little, wisdom comes with age because the old person has witnessed a wider range of the kinds of problems and the kinds of solutions which are effective in such a society. The greater adaptability possessed by the young affords them a distinct advantage over the conservatism and set ways of their elders in times of rapid change. Not only in adjustment to new means of production which may require learning new motor skills, but also in innovative management, marketing, executive roles, and research and development, the flexibility of youth is an asset. The heightened value of youth in these times of rapid change has provided the young with the economic independence to break ties with parents and elders who in a traditional agrarian society own the land, the sole source of livelihood. Furthermore, the wisdom of extensive experience, which in the static society of Hunza is justifiably highly prized in the elderly, loses its value in a rapidly changing society where the premium must be on adaptability rather than experience. The familiarity of an elder Hunzakut with weather and seasons that allows him to predict the optimal time for planting and harvesting, or the severity of the oncoming winter, is no match for modern weather forecasting. The latter is as available to the young as to the old and the wisdom of experience becomes redundant. Innovativeness and adaptability become the "wisdom" of the young, whereas, if the aged are less flexible, their rigidity may make them "unwise."

If the only means by which the elderly can achieve status and deserve respect is a return to an unchanging traditional society—a most unlikely prospect, today—then we would have to weigh the gains for the elders against the possible loss to the young. In a traditional stable society the extended family structure clearly provides benefits for the old, but what are the costs to the young? Decision-making remains the prerogative of the elderly, so there must be an associated limitation of choices for the young. But it is just the freedom to make their own decisions that motivates our youth to establish independent households. How restricted do the young (and even middle-aged) feel in traditional stable cultures? Do they rebel against a tyranny of their elders or do they accept this relation as in the nature of things, having known nothing different, and perhaps gain patience in the knowledge that in due time they will ascend to the status of their elders? There are clearly "cost benefits" to the individual and to society of social conditions which may favor respect for age versus freedom for youth. Can the one be had only at the expense of the other? Since there is little indication that society is likely spontaneously to return to stable traditional ways, it will take great ingenuity to develop conditions which will benefit both.

Retirement in our society is largely economically determined, and there seems to be no possibility of return to the agrarian existence of most of our forebears who lived in extended family groups. On the farm no one was too old to make some contribution to the social and economic life of the family. The chores might become less strenuous, but by performing them on a regular basis the elderly could always feel needed and useful.

It seems a corruption of the very purpose of our economy that,

instead of freeing us from drudgery and need and allowing us all
to enjoy a better life with the things it can produce, it holds us
slaves to its dictates even though affluence is at hand. We can
anticipate that continued automation of industry will bring
earlier retirement and shorter working hours. The devastating
effect of enforced leisure on the life span of the elderly and the
happiness of all could be countered in part by educational
programs. Such programs should have the purpose of arousing
interest and demonstrating the possibility of hobbies or avocations to which people can turn with zest when their contribution
to the industrial economy is no longer needed. The trend toward
shorter working hours and earlier retirement makes the need for
such education urgent. Creative activities such as music and the
arts, sports, and much-needed physical exercise, as well as crafts,
gardening, and many other interests, need active cultivation.
Involvement in services for less fortunate members of the
community, in protecting the environment, and in other such
socially constructive tasks can also be continued long after
retirement. Self-fulfillment in such pursuits can provide the
interest and joy of living that is so essential to a life-sustaining,
wholesome mental state.

The cultures of the three societies I visited provide for a strictly
male world. Women are subservient, doing all the household
menial work as well as helping their menfolk in the fields.
Enapshba Keskindzh, age 121, of Chloy, gave us his prescription
for a long life as "Go to the mountains—it is wonderful there."
He had married at forty-five years of age, and his wife, who is
twenty years younger than he, commented, "I kept him well by
working much harder than he, raising our seven children while
he went to the mountains as a shepherd and hunter." Particularly
the women, when asked what was the happiest period of their
lives, were not eager to turn back the clock to earlier years
because of the hard work they had had to endure. In Vilcabamba
the old people showed little *"joie de vivre."* When asked what she
remembers most vividly from her long life, Micaela Quezada, 102
years old, thought for a long while and said, "Nothing—all I
remember is hard work." This seemed typical of the responses in
Vilcabamba where life seems to go on with little change in a
pattern repeated day after day—work, sleep, procreate, and
eat—the routine being broken only by an occasional holiday
which meant a day off from work.

But we encountered no pessimists or hypochondriacs among

the elderly. Consistent with their feelings of security and important social role, they all seemed to take a very positive view of society and the future. There didn't even seem to be criticism of the new ways introduced by the young. Gregori Quokhia of Gulripshi, born January 10, 1871, thinks the modern generation is good and the world is fine. When pressed further he responded philosophically, "What isn't good I can't change anyway, so I don't worry about it." Many of the centenarians emphasized the importance of being independent and free to do the things they enjoyed and wanted to do and of maintaining a placid state of mind free from worry or emotional strain. "Now everywhere people don't live so long because they don't live a free life," commented Sonchka Kvetzenia, age 109, of Atara; "they worry more and don't do what they want. We worked less and lived poorer but we had more rest and were freer." Gabriel Chapnian, 117 years old, of Gulrepsh expressed a similar sentiment succinctly after reversing our roles and asking me if Americans live long. When told that few attain his age, he responded, "Hmm . . . too literate!"

In their remote farms and villages the old people I visited live largely oblivious to the pressures and strains of modern life. Such American concerns as the fighting in Southeast Asia, Watergate, conflict in the Middle East, starvation in Africa, genocide in Bangladesh, environmental pollution, the energy crisis, and the myriads of other disasters that fill our news media were unknown to them. In Vilcabamba we received only expressions of disbelief when we asked the villagers their reaction to the "moon walk." In Hunza even the words to ask such questions are lacking in the native tongue, Burashaski. In the Caucasus people were better informed about technological advances, but their agrarian existence, which was badly disturbed by World War II, has settled back to tranquility. The oft-repeated toast "To peace!" was a frequent reminder, however, that the ravages of the 1940s were not quickly forgotten.

Most of the stresses and tensions to which mankind is subject arise from more personal social interactions, such as a quarrel with a spouse or misbehavior by an offspring. As a result, it is impossible for members of any social group entirely to escape mental stress and tensions. Nonetheless, in societies that are less competitive and less aggressive even these personal stresses can be less frequent and less exhausting than they are in our own.

The role of emotional tensions and pressures on health and

longevity is not clearly understood. Common sense tells us that extremes of anger, fear, and hate do no good to our systems and may drive us to compulsive acts that may be life-threatening to ourselves or others. The extreme stimulation of our nervous systems under such circumstances may result in loss of consciousness or fainting from a fall in blood pressure and the loss of tone of small blood vessels or, at the other extreme, a severe spasm of blood vessels such as comes with hypertension from stimulation of the sympathetic nervous system. This latter state may cause such a strain on the heart as to precipitate angina or even a heart attack. Whether more chronic and unresolved nervous tensions can lead to sustained hypertension is not clear, though many believe this to be the case.

Just as there exists a personality type thought to be prone to develop peptic ulcer—the worrying, anxious person—so too there is a hypertensive stereotype. The overweight, overbearing, hard-driving, aggressive, tense, flushed middle-aged executive is the movie version of the hypertensive personality. However, the physical features need not be so obvious, and hypertension may become quite severe without one being aware of its presence. Since it can be treated effectively with medicines today it is one of the important reasons for regular checkups as part of preventive medical practice.

There have been several attempts to define the behavioral contribution to coronary heart disease. A "coronary-prone" behavior pattern has been described by R. H. Rosenman and his associates. The pattern, (Type A) is characterized by attributes such as hard-driving effort, striving for achievement, competitiveness, aggressiveness, haste, impatience, restlessness, alertness, uneven bursts of amplitude in speech, and hurried motor movements. Individuals with this pattern are usually conscientiously committed to their occupation and often have achieved success in it. This overt behavior pattern has been found to be associated with increased prevalence of coronary heart disease. By contrast, the Type B personality pattern is defined as essentially the converse of the Type A pattern. It is characterized by a relative absence of drive, ambition, sense of urgency, and the desire to compete or be involved in deadlines. The Type B pattern is considered to be infrequently associated with heart attacks.

Most of us will recognize some elements of the Type A pattern in ourselves. In fact, several features in the list are those we try to instill in our offspring and students—they are essential ingredients for "success" in our cultural ethic. Surely hard-driving effort and striving for achievement must be counted among the virtues which have built our national success. One senses here a conflict between societal benefits and our biological well-being, a conflict which becomes increasingly apparent as our world becomes more crowded.

In an attempt to assess the possible role of this behavior pattern in the development of coronary heart disease, Rosenman and his colleagues examined the relative importance of sociologic and behavior factors in coronary heart disease. Twelve social variables selected for study as possible precursors of coronary heart disease were the subject's country of birth, father's country of birth, mother's country of birth, father's religion, mother's religion, father's education, mother's education, father's occupation, subject's childhood residence, subject's education, subject's occupation and subject's income. The twelve biological variables also examined were: age, parental history of coronary heart disease, history of diabetes mellitus, cigarette smoking, the electrocardiogram, the coronary-prone behavior pattern (described in the preceding paragraph), obesity, systolic and diastolic blood pressure, serum total cholesterol, fasting triglycerides (the form in which the major neutral fats are present in the blood).

The 679 subjects who were selected for study were white male industrial employees, aged forty through forty-nine years at the start of the study in 1960–1961. Employed in banking, air transportation, aircraft manufacturing, and oil production in the San Francisco Bay area, the subjects are only a partially representative segment of the American industrial urban population. In 1966 the participants responded to a questionnaire constructed to evaluate the social factors listed and biological factors were assessed at annual examinations in that interval 1960 to 1967. During this period of observation thirty-seven subjects developed coronary heart disease.

When all twelve social factors were considered simultaneously, the key social variables were mother's religion, subject's education, father's religion, subject's income, and father's occupation. When the twelve standard biologic factors were considered simultaneously, the key biological variables were systolic blood pressure, age, cigarette smoking, serum cholesterol, and coronary-prone behavior. When these key social and biological variables were considered simultaneously, the most important social and biological discriminant variables were systolic blood pressure, the parental religion, age, serum cholesterol, cigarette smoking, father's occupation and the coronary-prone behavior. This analysis indicates that social factors as well as the standard biological risk factors were importantly related to the incidence of coronary heart disease.

In a recent prospective study the ability of the coronary-prone Type A behavior pattern measured by a computer-scored questionnaire to predict new coronary heart disease was tested: 2750 employed men ranging in age from forty-four to sixty-four years completed the questionnaire in 1965. All subjects were free of clinical coronary disease at that time. The study ended in 1969, by which time 120 subjects had clinical coronary heart disease. Those with high scores for coronary-prone Type A behavior pattern at the start of the study had twice the incidence of new coronary heart disease as low scorers over the four-year period of the study. In this study the scores on the questionnaire were unknown to the investigators who managed the follow-up study which determined the cases of new heart disease that had developed during the study. This technique protects against any conscious or unconscious bias in the results and lends credibility to the importance of psychological factors, as formulated by Rosenman and associates, as risk factors in the development of heart attacks.

There is a suggestion from statistical studies that a role for emotional tension in modifying longevity extends to occupational categories. In a comprehensive survey of mortality rates for males aged twenty to sixty-four years of age for the United States, England and Wales, H. King compared white males generally with physicians, lawyers, teachers, and white clergy. The mortality rates in the United States for the year 1950 from all causes were slightly less for all the learned professions than for the general male public, with teachers and clergy having lower rates than physicians and lawyers. However, when mortality rates from specific diseases were tabulated, physicians and lawyers were found to experience rates considerably in excess of white males generally for heart attacks. Lawyers were more subject to death from hypertension and physicians exceed other professions in suicides, whereas clergy have the lowest suicide rates. Mortality rates from diabetes were very high among physicians and clergy and cerebral vascular accidents claimed their highest toll from the same two professions. Clearly there is much social, economic, and even health selection in those who go into these professions, and it would be invalid to ascribe all the differences in mortality rates to occupation alone. These professionals represent a privileged class in our society in regard to education and economic and social status. Their long lives may be attributable to the consequences of these factors, perhaps in spite of the emotional tensions under which they may work and live.

In the three places I visited the old people generally adhere to a very fixed daily routine. Their lives are very ordered and regular. One schoolgirl in Abkhasia told us that they had no alarm clock in her house. "We don't need one because great Grandpa gets up at the same time every morning." They are creatures of habit. Smoking, eating, drinking, and sex all seem to be dealt with in moderation by the elderly—although we saw striking exceptions which illustrated that no single one of these was necessarily determinant of the life span. In this regard the Georgians like to tell the story of a centenarian who was visited and interviewed by a delegation on his one-hundred-fourteenth birthday. When asked to what he attributed his long life, he responded that he didn't smoke, he didn't drink, and he never chased women—to this he attributed his longevity. During the interview loud shouts, noises of a scuffle and a woman's screams were heard next door. This became so distracting that the delegates finally asked what the noise was all about. "Oh," said the centenarian, "don't pay any attention to that. It is only my older brother who always beats his sixth wife when he drinks too much."

Expectations of longevity may also be important. In contrast to the "three score and ten" which most young Americans would provide as an answer, the young people of Abkhasia generally responded to our question of how long they expected to live by saying "to a hundred." Dr. Gyorgi Kaprashvili of Gulripshi confirmed that the public has the notion that the normal life span of man is 100 years. For exaggeration when proposing toasts they may say 300 years, but everyone expects to be 100. Perhaps our expectations are too limited and we program our lives to a shorter existence accordingly.

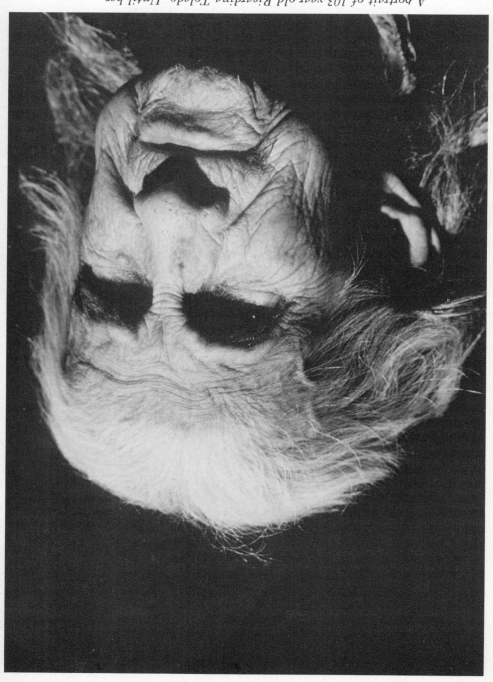

A portrait of 103-year-old Ricardina Toledo. Until her retirement seven years ago, she worked hard in the fields.

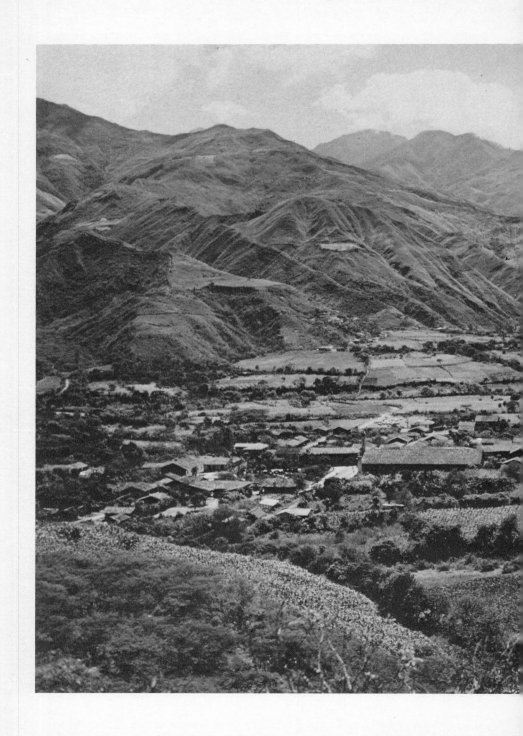

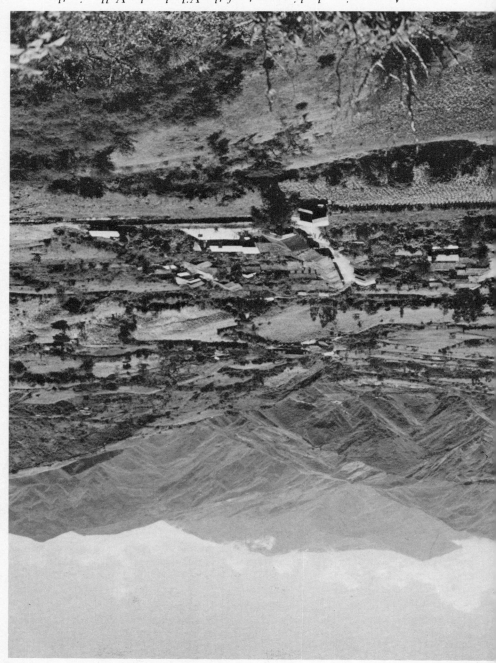

An overview, looking west, of the Vilcabamba Valley in the foothills of the Ecuadorian Andes.

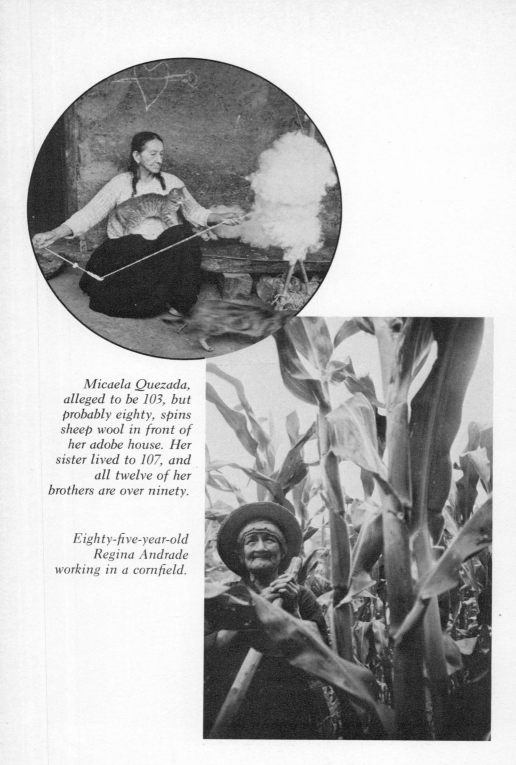

Micaela Quezada, alleged to be 103, but probably eighty, spins sheep wool in front of her adobe house. Her sister lived to 107, and all twelve of her brothers are over ninety.

Eighty-five-year-old Regina Andrade working in a cornfield.

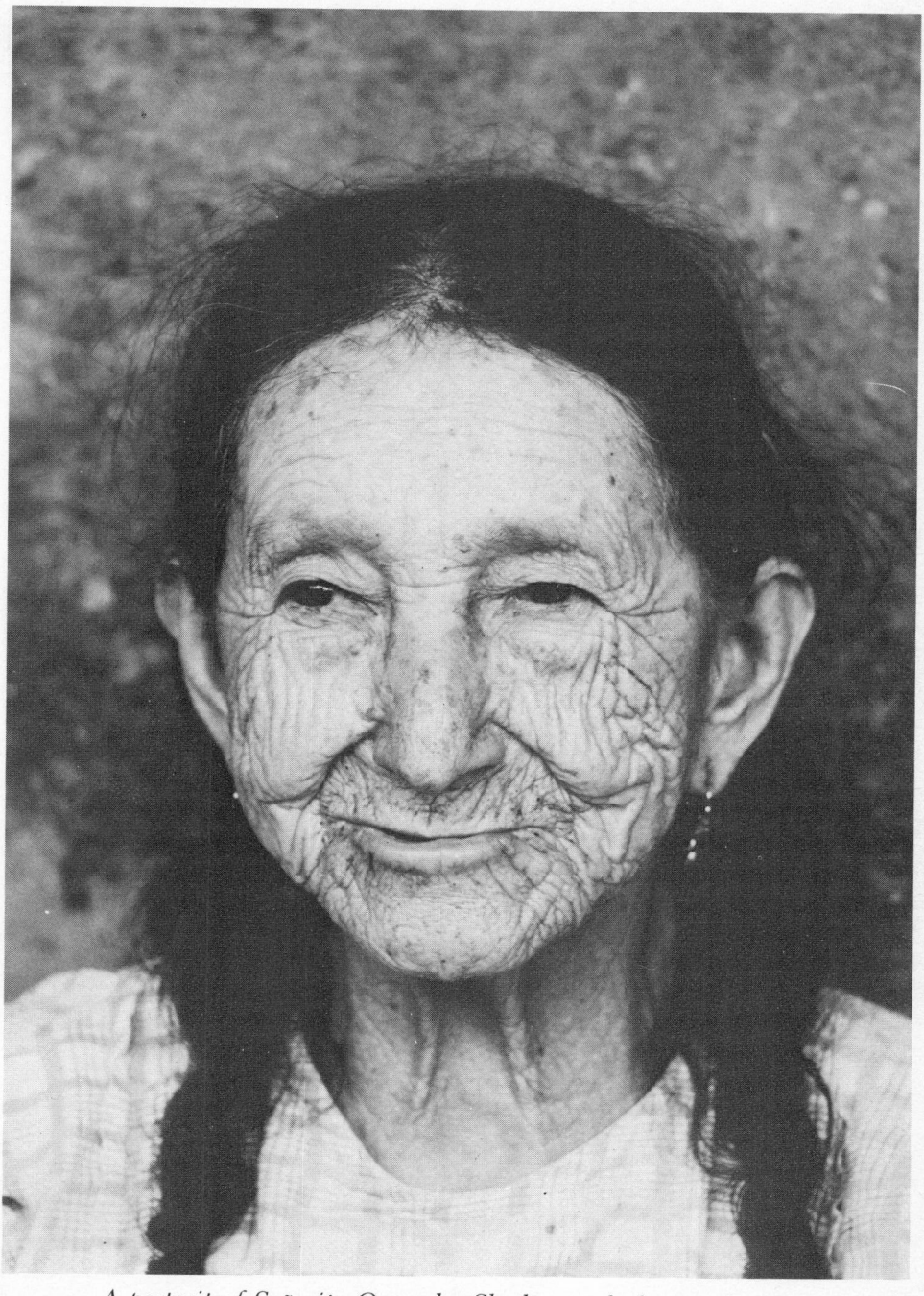

A portrait of Señorita Quezada. She has worked every day of her adult life. She does not drink or smoke, but she thoroughly enjoys her five cups of South American coffee a day.

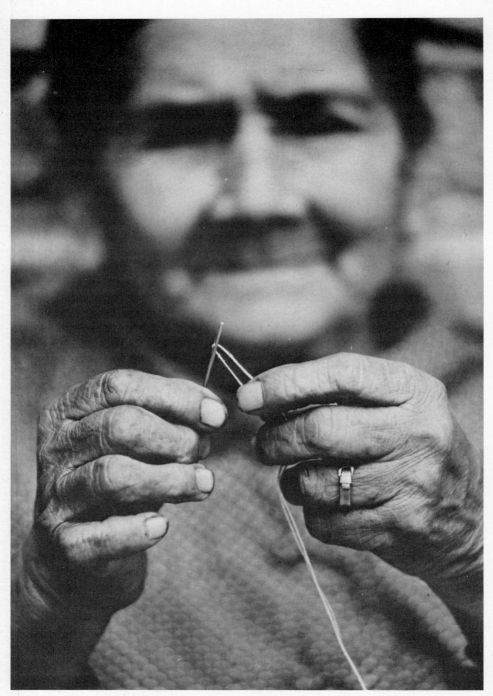

Señora Clodovea Herrera, 103, threading a needle.

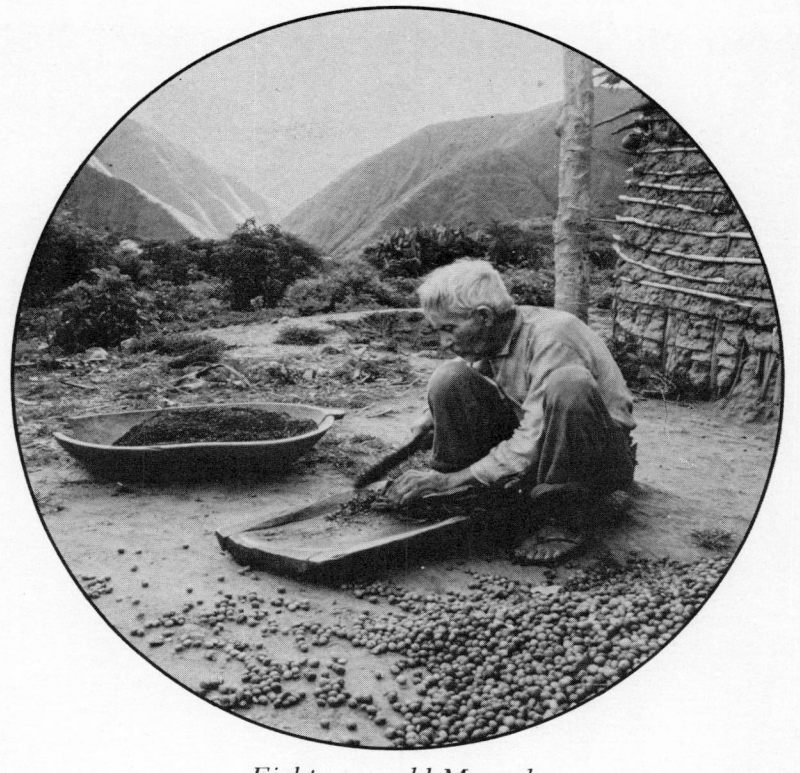

Eighty-year-old Manuel Armijos works cutting tobacco leaves.

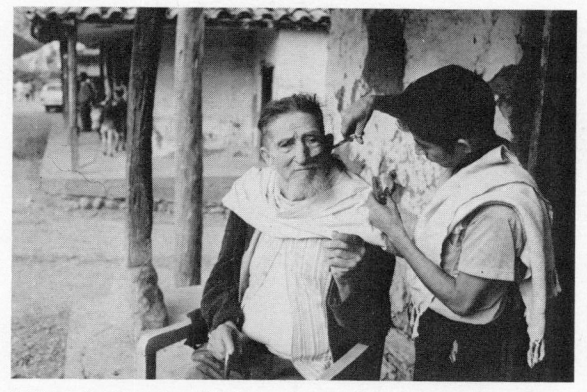

Miguel Carpio, believed to be 123, but probably not more than 110, has his hair cut. Until he was almost sixty years old he hunted sheep in the steep Andean foothills. Señor Carpio would not like to be young again, but he said, "If I could take fifteen years from my age—wonderful!"

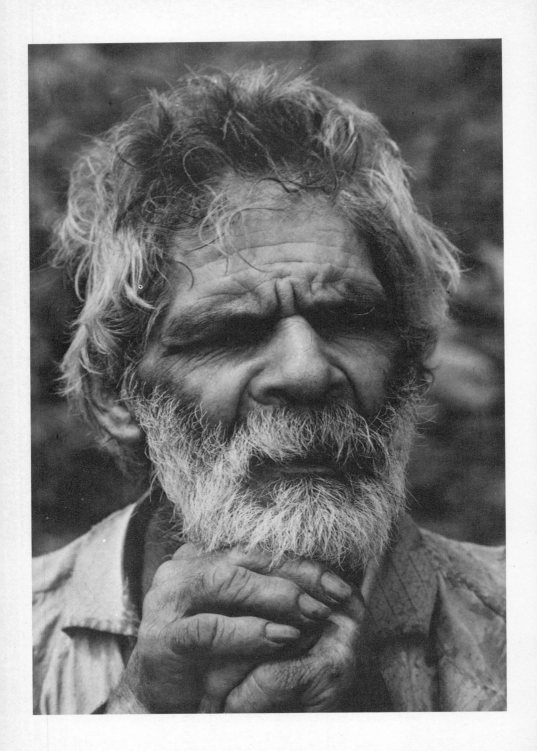

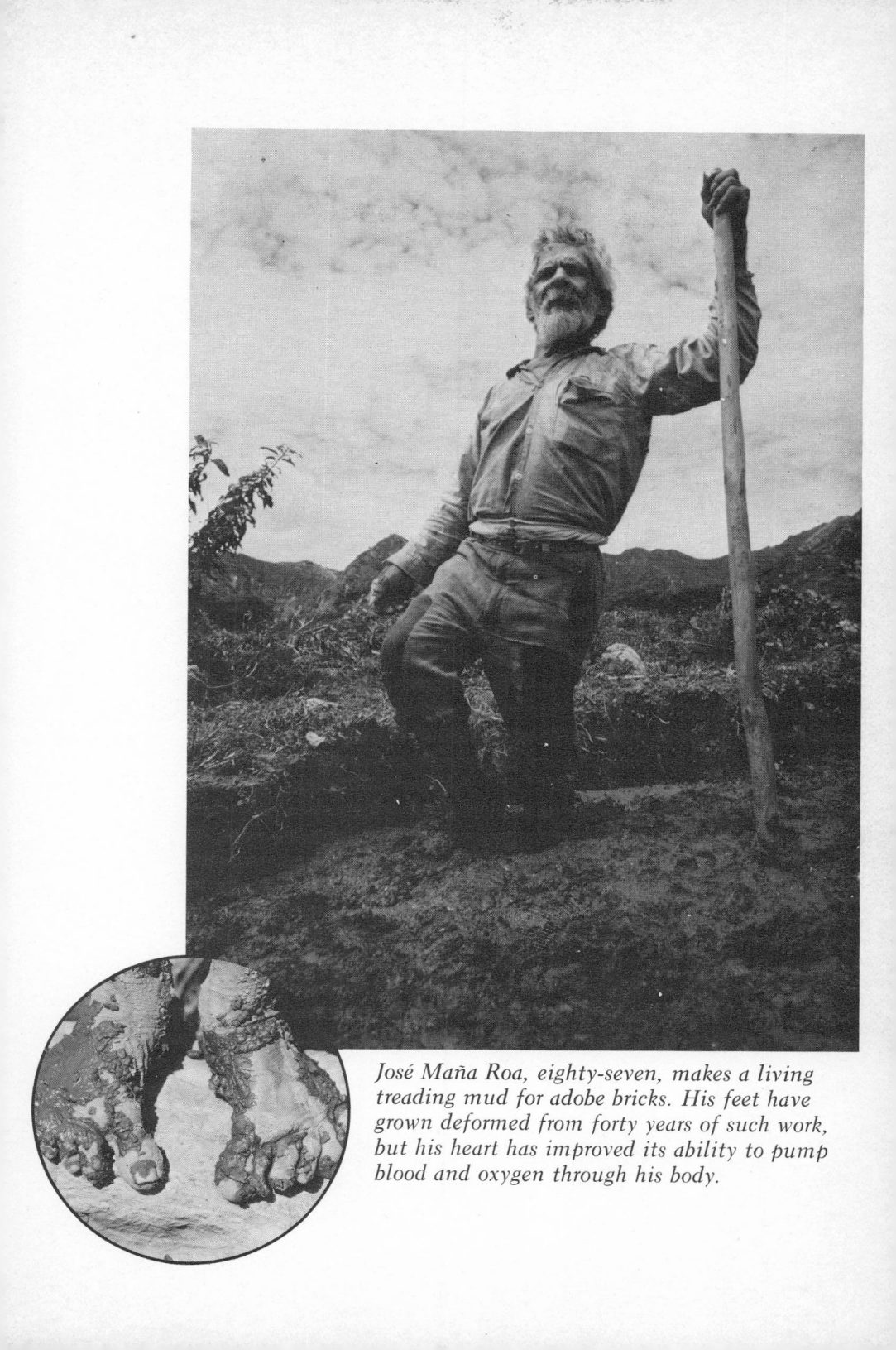

José Maña Roa, eighty-seven, makes a living treading mud for adobe bricks. His feet have grown deformed from forty years of such work, but his heart has improved its ability to pump blood and oxygen through his body.

11

RESEARCH IN AGING

The society which fosters research to save human life cannot escape responsibility for the life thus extended. It is for science not only to add years to life but, more important, to add life to the years.

George M. Piersol (1880–1966) and Edward L. Bortz (1896–1970), *Annals of Internal Medicine*, 12:964, 1939.

In spite of millennia of speculations—some subdued but some quite wild—regarding the causes, nature, and meaning of aging, a scientific probing into the problem has occurred only recently. Many fascinating questions about the molecular and cellular basis of aging can now be asked and answers sought through application of modern scientific methods. The field is opening up and the stigmata of charlatanism and pseudoscience that have so long cast their shadows over anyone professing interest in the subject are yielding to the application of rigorous science. Scientists who work in this area are referred to as gerontologists; gerontology is the study of aging. Geriatricians, by contrast, are physicians or therapists who treat the ills of old age; geriatrics is the branch of medicine which deals with the ailments of the elderly.

It is thought that, if one were to strip away disease states, including heart attacks, strokes, and cancer, there would still remain an aging process that would decrease the adaptability of the individual to survive the vicissitudes in his environment until death finally supervened. The tendency today is to believe that there is mortality even without disease—or, stated another way, aging is a normal universal process rather than an accumulation of lesions which should be regarded as pathological. Whether a given change in structure or function is regarded as part of a normal universal process or pathological often becomes a moot issue and the discussions at this point become philosophical and semantic.

Is there an absolute limit to the life span of man? If so, what determines the limit? What is it that makes cells or organisms age? What are the individual biochemical and molecular changes whose sum total constitutes the aging process? Are these changes irrevocable consequences of the genetic information contained in each cell, or do they result from the cumulative effects of repeated, nonlethal injuries to which a hostile environment repeatedly subjects all living matter? These are the questions now being asked by scientists in laboratories in many countries. It will be answers to these questions which will determine the possibility and feasibility of extending the natural life span. The advisability of so doing will remain another major question.

I would like to give you a glimpse—though of necessity brief, incomplete, and superficial—of the approaches currently under investigation. If the reader concludes that this field is still in a rudimentary, groping stage, most gerontologists would agree. It is only with the advances in molecular and cellular biology of the last twenty years that studies of various mechanisms have become possible. Prior to that only descriptive data cataloguing the changes in various systems with aging were collected and even that phase of study remains incomplete.

Although there is some increase in size through enlargement of individual cells, growth occurs in the human primarily through multiplication of cells by cell division. In the adult cell, division, however, continues, but at a rate which just replaces cells which have died. A steady state of individual and of organ size is maintained by replenishing cells which die through division of remaining cells and differentiation of the new daughter cells to the mature cell type being replaced. The rate of cell death and replacement of dead cells varies greatly from one tissue or organ to another. As indicated earlier, nerve cells of the brain do not partake of such a turnover in the adult; a nerve cell lost from whatever cause in the adult brain cannot be replaced. Cells lining the small intestine, on the other hand, are shed and lost into the bowel at a high rate such that their average survival is only one or two days. The process of replenishing these intestinal cells continues throughout adult life but the turnover may slow with age.

Even cells which are not replaceable, however, are not static during their life. Nerve cells of the brain and other nerve cells are continuously building and degrading their constitutent parts. During the life of the cell it is probable that every molecule comprising the cell, with the exception of DNA, may be degraded and replaced not once but many times. The degree of this turnover is often astounding. In a recent study it has been demonstrated that the urinary bladder accommodates to filling not only by stretching and flattening of the cells which comprise its inner lining, but there also occurs a simultaneous synthesis of considerable amounts of new cell surface membranes. This serves to expand the surface of the bladder and its retentive capacity. With emptying of the bladder the cell membranes are excessive for the contracted state and the surplus membranes are promptly degraded. This process of synthesis and degradation goes on continuously helping to accommodate the size of the organ to its functional state. The atrophy or shrinkage of muscles which are not used and their increase in girth with exercise is another familiar example of this turnover of cell constituents. But this is only an obvious example of a process which goes on in an invisible, more subtle form in all cells throughout their life span.

If cells which cannot be replenished in adult life did not die, and if those that are replenishable were replaced with perfect copies of those lost, aging would not occur. The aging process, as it affects the intact individual, must be explicable in terms of understanding what causes deterioration and depopulation of nonreplenishing cell types, such as brain and heart cells, and what causes failure of replenishable cell types to replicate themselves perfectly and in sufficient numbers to keep pace with the continuous attrition of their kind.

Possible explanations for the process of aging may thus be sought at each level of organization of living matter: at the molecular, the cellular, the organ, and finally at the level of the overall regulation of the entire body. Undoubtedly changes at each level will occur and aging of the individual, as we recognize it, will be the sum total of these involutionary changes which will proceed at quite variable rates in the different cells, tissues, and organs of different individuals. First, I will consider the current state of understanding of molecular changes with aging.

MOLECULAR AGING

The mapping of the structure of the genetic material, deoxyribonucleic acid (DNA), made possible the great advances in molecular and cellular biology of the past twenty years. The genetic message is written according to the sequence in which four nucleotide bases are linked together to form the long threadlike molecules of DNA contained within the nucleus of our cells. Two of these long DNA strands are joined as complementary pairs and each pair is twisted together to form a double helix. "Reading" of the genetic message consists of separation of the two strands of DNA and the synthesis of complementary molecules of RNA (ribonucleic acid) which are comprised again of four nucleotide bases each designated by a specific nucleotide base in the parent DNA. The order or sequence of the four specific bases within the DNA thus determine the sequence of complementary bases within the RNA. Since the latter in turn code for specific amino acids, an assembly of amino acids along the length of the RNA molecules results in the synthesis of specific proteins. These are the proteins which comprise the enzymes and structural molecules of our bodies. Furthermore, the assemblage of the specific sequence and the linking together of the nucleotide bases of DNA and of RNA, as well as the linking together of the constituent amino acids into proteins, are accomplished via the activity of a host of specific enzymes, which, like all enzymes, are proteins. These enzymes in turn are coded for, read out, and synthesized in the manner just described.

In summary, the genetic message contained in DNA is first transcribed into specific RNA molecules which in turn determine the specific proteins which are the major structural and functional molecules of our bodies. It is in some step or steps within this complex cascade of critical chemical reactions that most gerontologists believe errors may arise which to a greater or lesser extent introduce "noise" and garble the translation of the genetic message. Whether such error is programmed into the original genetic message—"programmed" senescence—and thus inevitable, or whether it results from an accumulation of environmentally induced errors and hence potentially avoidable, remains a crucial but unanswered question.

Alterations in the synthesis of DNA, RNA, or proteins are likely causes of the aging process. Damage to RNA or proteins involved in synthesis of cell components may result in faulty molecules which compromise the viability of cells. Although the cell has mechanisms for repairing damage or compensating for it, some errors might occur in molecules in which the effect is self-reinforcing. An error, for example, in the sequence of one RNA molecule, which serves as a template to direct the synthesis of many identical protein molecules, might turn out inactive enzyme molecules from its production line. Probably every enzyme is subject to structural mutations which may range from no effect on function of the enzymes to the lowest level of function compatible with life. If the function of the enzyme is necessary for the life of the cell, once the enzyme has been mutated beyond usefulness the cell will die.

L. E. Orgel has suggested that certain enzymes involved in the transcription of information from DNA may deteriorate with aging so that incorrect messages are read out. This would lead to a self-reinforcing effect which would result in an "error catastrophe" and death of the cell. The consequences of this hy-

FIGURE 2
Protein Synthesis:
a. *In the nucleus,* unwinding of the double helix of DNA allows the genetic message to be transcribed in the synthesis of complementary messenger RNA.

b. *In the cytoplasm,* the messenger RNA is processed through a ribosome which translates the genetic message of the RNA into new protein. Amino acids are brought to the ribosomes by specific Transfer factors and assembled in the ribosome into new protein according to the instructions coded into the structure of the messenger RNA.

PROTEIN SYNTHESIS

a. IN THE NUCLEUS

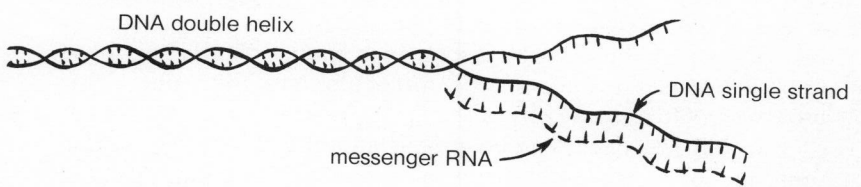

DNA double helix

DNA single strand

messenger RNA

b. IN THE CYTOPLASM

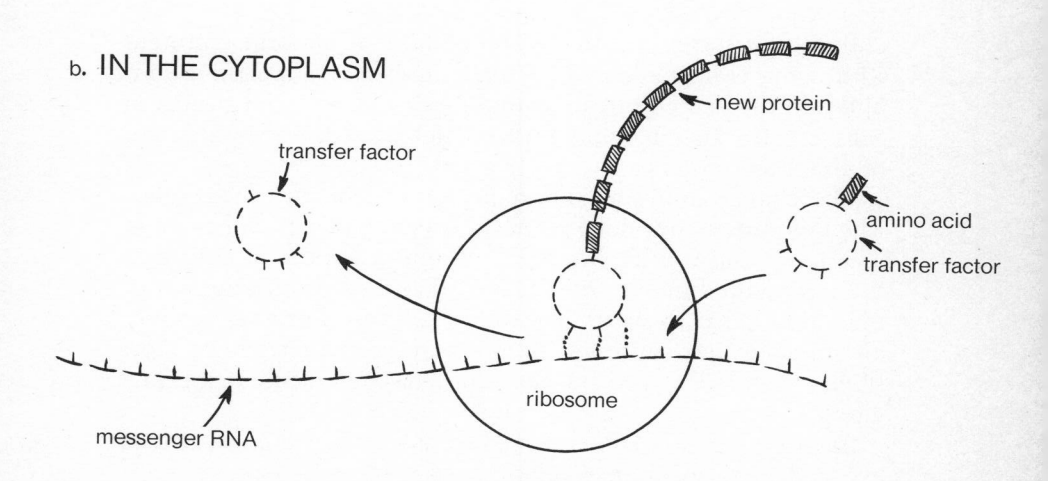

new protein

transfer factor

amino acid

transfer factor

ribosome

messenger RNA

pothesis, that aged cells would synthesize more faulty proteins than young cells, has been tested; results at present largely support Orgel's hypothesis.

It is possible to test the homogeneity of enzyme molecules by several means. One way is to measure the activity of the enzyme at increasing temperatures. Heating will inactivate enzymes. If all the enzyme molecules are identical they will all be inactivated at the same temperature. However, if the enzyme molecules differ even slightly, then some will be inactivated at a lower temperature and others perhaps at a higher temperature than the norm. In this latter case there will occur a gradual inactivation of the enzymatic activity as the temperature is increased.

Studies have been conducted on the effect of heat inactivation of enzymes isolated from young and aging cell cultures. When glucose-6-phosphate dehydrogenase—a key enzyme in the utilization of glucose—isolated from young cultures of fibroblasts, is heated, enzymatic activity decays in a manner indicative of a homogeneous enzyme; all the molecules are the same. The enzyme isolated from cells in the late senescent stage of culture, on the contrary, decays on heating in a manner which reveals the presence of considerable abnormal enzyme protein. Similar results have been demonstrated with other enzymes; the proportion of inactive enzyme molecules increases with the age of the culture. Furthermore, the accumulation of abnormal protein with aging is dependent upon the number of population doublings in the cell cultures; treatments which arrest the growth of cells, e.g. freezing in liquid nitrogen, delay also the accumulation of abnormal proteins.

The change in an enzyme molecule which will cause diminished or absent enzymatic (catalytic) activity may be very subtle. The exact and specific sequence of amino acids is so critical to the enzymatic function of a protein that a single substitution of one amino acid by another in the chain of a hundred or more amino acids may cause loss of enzymatic activity while by most other criteria the protein molecule has not been detectably altered.

Agents which are known to induce errors of protein synthesis age cell cultures prematurely. This occurs in association with increased abnormal enzyme proteins in the cells. The cellular machinery makes proteins, as has been discussed, by hooking together naturally occurring amino acids into long, thread-like chains, which then fold spontaneously into the protein molecule.

172

By adding abnormal, man-made amino acids into the culture medium, the cell may be tricked into incorporating these abnormal amino acids into new proteins being made. When this is done the cell cultures undergo premature aging. Treatments which cause abnormal proteins to be made in the cell by scrambling the order of normal, natural-occurring amino acids within a protein will also accelerate cell aging in culture. Causing the synthesis of abnormal proteins in cells thus hastens the aging process, and the aging process as it occurs in dividing cell cultures is associated with the spontaneous accumulation of abnormal proteins in the cells. These observations would seem to show a close relationship between the presence of abnormal proteins and the aging process, but whether the relationship is a causal one requires further investigation.

One ingenious study took advantage of the known fact that viruses, when they infect cells, preempt the protein-making machinery of the host cells to produce proteins necessary for the growth and multiplication of new viruses. In this study aged culture cells, when infected with virus, supported replication of the virus as well as did young cells. This is evidence, in this instance, at least, that the protein-synthesizing mechanism of the old cells was operating without detectable increased error. This observation represents a special case and may not contradict the generality of the Orgel hypothesis.

Z. Medvedev, a prominent Russian student of the biology of aging, has postulated "active aging" due to genes which become activated at a predetermined stage in life. These genes purposefully introduce "noise" or error into the synthetic machinery and shorten the life of the cell. This programmed obsolescence would act in addition to the spontaneous mutagenic factors acting on somatic cells and hasten the demise of the organism, preventing thereby accumulation of deleterious mutations in germ cells which would eventually prove lethal to the species.

F. M. Burnet accepts that somatic mutations (affecting body cells in contrast to the germ cells) is the primary means by which aging is mediated and suggests that the link connecting the somatic changes with the genetic material is that the rate of somatic mutation in any mammal is under genetic control and operates through the structure of the enzymes responsible for insuring the fidelity of DNA duplication. Accurate duplication of DNA, which must occur when cells divide, is not wholly due to the complementarity of the nucleotide base pairs, but requires also the action of DNA polymerase and other enzymes which assemble and connect the individual nucleotide bases in proper order to form the DNA. These polymerases, in turn, being proteins, must be under genetic control. So-called "mutator genes" have been demonstrated in lower forms and may increase the rate of mutations through their control of the synthesis of DNA polymerase. Rates of mutation may exceed the expectation from environmental sources—ionizing radiation or chemical mutagens—as a result of the alterations in DNA polymerase. For species that must adapt rapidly to changing or different environments such heightened mutation rates in the germ cells will serve to accelerate the process of natural selection. In somatic cells mutations would produce the changes associated with cell aging.

Thus far I have considered the accumulation of "error molecules" in the aging cell as due solely to mistakes in synthesis. It has been known that, during the life of a cell, its content of proteins and other molecules, excepting perhaps only its DNA, are in a dynamic state. That is, a continuous synthesis and degradation of most molecules goes on, and the content of any cell constituent at one point in time depends on the balance between rates of synthesis and of degradation of that constituent. There is thus a continuous turnover of molecules comprising the cell throughout the life of the cell. Just as cells that make up the skin which covers our bodies continuously die and are replaced by new skin cells, maintaining an intact integument, so too are the molecules which make up the individual cells "turning over" during the life of the cell. Furthermore, the rate of turnover of different molecules within a single cell varies greatly. The turnover of proteins has been most extensively studied and the life span of different proteins within cells may vary from a few minutes to months. Even within a single cell large variation will exist in the "life span" of different protein molecules.

In general, studies reveal that abnormal proteins synthesized within cells are destroyed or degraded more rapidly than normal proteins. A failure of the degradative process within old cells could lead to the accumulation of "error proteins" just as might mistakes in synthesis. Today we have very little understanding of how cells remove abnormal molecules which may arise with time from natural wear and tear of cellular constituents or from mistakes in synthesis that arise from somatic mutations. Research in this direction is only commencing but promises to be of importance. Our ignorance of this basic process points up again the need for much further research to increase our understanding of the process of aging.

The DNA which carries the genetic information is provided with repair systems in the nuclei of cells. These repair systems will mend breaks or inappropriate attachments between nucleic acids within a single strand of the double-stranded DNA. Such breaks or adhesions may result from irradiation of the cell either by the continuous bombardment of cosmic rays or exposure to X rays or ultraviolet irradiation. Enzymes in the nucleus can excise the damaged portion of the strand and other enzymes, DNA polymerases, will then replace the appropriate purine and pyrimidine bases to realign with the complementary bases in the adjoining portion of the intact strand of DNA. In this manner the error is corrected, the double-stranded DNA of the normal cell is reconstituted and the genetic message preserved. Presumably, when the rate of damage to the DNA exceeds the ability to repair the damage, then faulty information enters the genetic message and it becomes garbled. Misrepair may also garble the message.

The importance of DNA repair mechanisms have been shown in progeria, a condition associated with premature aging. J. Epstein and associates found that fibroblasts from a subject with progeria, when grown in cell culture, cannot repair breaks in DNA produced by heavy X-radiation. Similar damage in normal cells is completely repaired within thirty minutes. This condition indicates that serious problems for preservation of normal cell growth arise when mechanisms for repairing DNA injury are defective. Then environmental factors—X ray or ultraviolet rays, in the examples cited—can produce changes which in the progeria case, at least, mimics senescence.

Many of the effects of exposure to X rays (gamma rays) are similar to the process of aging. However, the shortened life span of animals and humans exposed to excessive radiation is due almost entirely to an increased incidence of cancer. Also, the changes induced by exposure to X rays even in doses which shorten life are not accompanied by the increased crosslinking of collagen molecules which invariably is associated with natural aging. Irradiation thus may be a potent means of introducing mutational damage into the genetic material of dividing and nondividing somatic cells, but the results do not seem identical with the process of aging, perhaps because of other effects of X rays such as on the immune system.

H. P. von Hahn, and subsequently other investigators, have

reported that DNA obtained from old animals undergoes dena-
turation at higher temperatures than is the case with DNA from
younger animals of the same species. This suggests stronger
intermolecular bonding in the DNA from old animals. He also
found that histones—the small basic proteins which bind to the
acidic nucleic acids—were more tightly bound to the DNA from
old animals than was the case with DNA from young animals.
These effects would serve to stabilize the DNA double helix
preventing the two strands from unwinding and hence from
transcribing RNA. Without transcribing its genetic message to
RNA, protein synthesis would diminish, essential enzymes would
no longer be replaced, and the cell would die. The stronger
intermolecular binding between DNA strands and between DNA
and histones might result from spontaneous cross-linking reactions which increased with time.

One highly reproducible finding with age has been the increased intermolecular cross-linking and reduced solubility of
collagen. Collagen is the protein elaborated by fibroblasts which
is the major structural constituent of our bodies; it makes up
connective tissue, tendons, the organic matrix of bone, and
generally holds us together. It constitutes also some thirty
percent of the protein in our bodies. With aging there occurs a
continuous increase in spontaneous cross-linking of neighboring
fibers of collagen. This stiffens and rigidifies our tissues. The
increase in cross-linking is so constant with time that its degree
has been proposed as an objective means to estimate the chronological age of a subject. It was thought at one time that the
increased stiffening of blood vessels due to cross-linking of the
collagen molecules in their walls might impede blood flow
through the vessel and decrease nutrition of cells and tissues,
with the eventual loss of some cells. However, though this
macromolecular cross-linking does occur, few believe it to be the
primary cause of the aging process. It apparently is not known
whether in conditions associated with accelerated senescence
(such as progeria or Werner's syndrome) there is also an accelerated rate of cross-linking of collagen.

Free radicals (atoms or molecules having at least one unpaired
electron and as a consequence possessing high chemical reactivity), formed in our bodies by chemical reactions or by irradiation
and have long been known to cause oxidative damage to molecules and to cells. They may cause oxidative alterations in the
long-lived macromolecules comprising the chromosomal or ge-

netic material. In this way they may act as mutagenic agents. They also cause breakdown of cell membranes, of mucin, and of other biologically important molecules. They may result in accumulation within cells of inert materials such as lipofuscin which arise from oxidative polymerization reactions involving largely polyunsaturated fats. Lipofuscin may accumulate in such large amounts within nerve cells of the brain as to cause a loss of cell function. Because of the deleterious effects of free radicals and their possible causal role in the aging process, studies have been conducted by D. Harman, R. R. Kohn, and others to determine if the feeding of antioxidants to animals will delay senescence. In the experiments of Harman with mice the mean life span was extended modestly, but there was no extension of the maximal life span. Furthermore, mixing the antioxidants he tested with the food resulted in weight loss of his animals due to decreased food intake, which itself is known to extend the life span of mice. Vitamin E, which is the normal antioxidant we ingest in our diets, has not been found to extend the life span of experimental animals.

CELLULAR AGING

At the cellular level, studies of aging have been given a big boost by the experiments of Leonard Hayflick of Stanford University, who has examined cell survival in cell cultures. Methods for culturing cells and tissues in the laboratory have developed since the beginning of this century with great improvements in these techniques in recent years. Hayflick found that normal fibroblast cells—cells that form connective tissue and tendons—obtained from human embryos, when grown in tissue culture, undergo approximately 50 ± 10 divisions (population doublings) and then spontaneously die out.

This exciting finding has now been confirmed in several different laboratories and the observations extended. The number of doublings *in vitro* of fibroblasts obtained by biopsy of human skin was found to be inversely related to the age of the donor—the older the subject the fewer cell divisions before the cells died out. Statistical analysis indicates a decrement of 0.20 population doublings per year of donor life in cultured human fibroblasts. This study included biopsies of skin from the inner aspect of the upper arm in 100 subjects ranging from fetal to ninety years of age. Thus fibroblasts grown from the bit of skin of the ninety-year-old would undergo some eighteen fewer doublings in culture than the fifty doublings characteristic of fetal tissue.

Furthermore, if the doubling of cells was interrupted for variable periods by immersing the cultures in liquid nitrogen (a procedure which halts biological action), on thawing the frozen cells would resume their dividing and complete the remainder of the fifty doublings before dying out. Others have shown that delaying or stopping cell divisions by omitting nutrients from the incubating medium may greatly protract survival. When such cells were returned to a proliferative state (resume dividing) by placing them in normal growth medium, they achieved cell divisions equal in number to control cells which had been continuously cultured on adequate growth medium. The finite life span of these normal human cells was related to the number of cumulative doublings rather than the calendar time in culture. This experiment in cell culture is almost the equivalent of the nutritional studies in the whole animal by C. M. McCay, who prolonged the life span of laboratory rats by providing a calorie-deficient diet which retarded their growth.

Embryo fibroblasts from other species also have been reported to undergo a finite number of doublings *in vitro*. This figure ranged from five to thirty-five population doublings for fibroblasts from chick embryo and fourteen to twenty-eight for mouse and thirty for marsupial fibroblasts. Man, with the longest life span among the warm blooded animals, has the largest number of doublings *in vitro* of normal fibroblast compared to any other species tested thus far. Of course, not all cell types from the same species necessarily have the capacity to undergo the same number of divisions. Nerve cells, which never undergo division once their quota in the brain is achieved, must have a different potential for replication than the cells lining the small intestine, for example, which slough off every twenty-four to forty-eight hours throughout the life of the individual. Only when comparing a specific cell type in one species to another can species differences in doubling ability be ascertained.

Hayflick's studies support the notion that a limited doubling potential is a characteristic of normal human and animal cells. Only cancer cells seem capable of eternal life in cell culture studies. One familiar line of cancer cells, the "HeLa" strain, has often been used in laboratory studies; it originated as a cervical cancer twenty-three years ago and has been maintained in culture ever since. Other strains of human cancer cells have been kept growing and multiplying continuously in culture for over sixty years. Clearly an understanding of what event or change occurred in these transformed (cancer) cells to release them from the bondage of mortality would contribute enormously to the understanding of the problem of cancer and of longevity.

Not all gerontologists accept Hayflick's experimental findings. The possibility has been suggested that the culture media might not indefinitely supply the fastidious growth requirements of normal mammalian cells; some trace substances required for growth may be exhausted, or lethal factors accumulate. This has been countered by the repeated changes of media that are employed and the fact that strains of cancer cells will survive indefinitely in the same media. A very elegant experiment by Hayflick excludes the action of some toxic substance in the medium as responsible for the limited doublings. He mixed cultures of fibroblasts obtained originally from male and female fetuses. The XX chromosome of the female, which is readily detected microscopically, was utilized as a cell marker to identify the female cells. The fibroblasts from the male fetus after forty replications in culture were mixed with an equal number of younger female fibroblasts which had been cultured only through ten doublings. If inadequacy of the culture medium or accumulation of a toxic factor were the primary causes of cell death, then in this experiment all cells should have expired at the same time after mixing the cells; a nutritional deficiency or toxic factor would not be expected to distinguish between a male or a female fibroblast. Actually, the male cells lived out their expected ten additional doublings while the female cells survived much longer, completing the expected forty further doublings. Studies of this kind have shown unambiguously that the finite life span of the cultured cells was an intrinsic property of the cells and not the effect of the culture media.

But normal body cells never grow in isolation. They grow, live, and function in conjunction and in harmony with many other types of cells in the body interchanging chemical messages continuously with them. Perhaps it is the deprivation of this "social" contact which ultimately leads to the demise of normal cells in culture. However, the equivalent of the Hayflick experiment has been performed in the whole animal by A. R. Williamson and B. A. Askonas. These investigators selected a single antibody-forming cell clone (group of cells originating through cell division of a single ancestor cell and thus all possessing identical genes) and propagated it by serial transfer to a limited number of spleen cells into irradiated genetically identical mice. Original spleen cell donors were immunized to a specific antigen. A single clone was identified by its characteristic secreted antibody to the specific antigen. Using this antibody as a cell marker it was possible to follow one clone of antibody forming cells through successive transfers from one mouse to the next. Recipients of spleen cells containing the specific antibody-forming cells consistently exhibited the characteristic antibody molecules in their sera. Sera of recipients of the eighth transfer contained only traces or lacked the characteristic antibodies, indicating that the specific antibody forming cell line had died out. Senescence and extinction of the cell line was estimated to have occurred after approximately ninety cell divisions. Other *in vivo* studies with mammary tissue, skin, and blood cells have come to similar conclusions. Thus a finite number of cell divisions would seem to be the case in the live animal just as Hayflick has demonstrated in cell culture.

There have been questions raised as to the applicability of Hayflick's findings to all normal mammalian cells. Do they all have a finite life in cell culture? Mouse cells, some claim, will live indefinitely. Whether these have undergone transformation by viruses or other agents and are behaving like cancer cells is likely, but not yet clearly established.

Further studies utilizing the cell culture techniques of Hayflick have been performed on tissues from humans with a variety of conditions known to shorten life expectancy. These studies suggested some increased rate of senescence in cultures from diabetics and prediabetic subjects as compared with fibroblasts from age matched normal subjects. Progeria, a condition characterized by accelerated aging, in which death from heart attacks occur in the small wizened gnomelike patients at the age of eight to twelve years, has given mixed results on cell culture. One study reported very few cell doublings in culture, but another revealed only a moderate decrease. Both showed, however, poor growth activity of progeria cells in culture. Werner's syndrome, another genetic condition characterized by premature aging, showed a definite decrease in the number of cell replications.

Interesting and fundamental as such studies are, they do not prove that the death of the individual is determined by the ultimate exhaustion of potential for cell division. Hayflick has stated that the likelihood is small that the animal dies because one or more important cell populations lose their proliferative capacity. He thinks it more likely that other changes or functional losses which have been demonstrated to accumulate in cells as they age may limit life before the cell line exhausts its potential to divide. Also these studies do not yet resolve, as Hayflick points out, whether the loss of potential for further cell division is an intrinsic part of the genetic program contained within each cell or whether it is attributable to cumulative damage to information-containing molecules during the life of the cell.

These studies do establish a model for the study of senescence in isolated cell cultures, and it is of obvious interest to the gerontologist to ascertain why the normal cell line dies out on repeated culture. As cell cultures approach their limiting number of divisions the time interval for cell doubling increases progressively, there is a gradual cessation of mitotic activity, fewer cells will divide, cellular debris accumulates, and finally total loss of vigor and death of the culture occurs. These degenerative phenomena manifest themselves after about fifty cell population doublings in the case of human embryo fibroblasts. What are the changes within the cells that cause their senescence with repeated doublings?

Not much is yet known of the biochemical events associated with this senescence. There is no accompanying change in oxygen consumption or glucose utilization, but more subtle changes are being found. Synthesis of DNA (the molecules which carry the genetic information) is reduced and occurs in only some of the cells, and synthesis of RNA (which follows from DNA) continues but at a reduced level. The senescent cells are larger than cells of earlier generations. There is an increased amount of lysosomal enzymes in these senescent cells, the enzymes which serve to scavenge and digest cellular debris. Other proteins are synthesized less rapidly, but changes in the synthesis and metabolism of lipids and other constituents of cells have not been adequately examined.

A very recent report from the laboratory of Leslie Packer at Berkeley indicates that addition of vitamin E to the culture medium of one strain of human fibroblasts has extended the number of population doublings to over one hundred, with no growth deterioration or microscopic evidence of senescence.

This important and fascinating finding needs confirmation and proof that the cell line has not undergone transformation to a malignant state. If true, it will provide the evidence that the heretofore observed limit of some fifty population doublings was not genetically predetermined but, in fact, due to an accumulation of environmental damage, presumably from free radicals.

A very promising approach to the study of aging is through the immune system. R. L. Walford and others have shown that with increasing age there occurs a diminution in the immune response to foreign proteins. But, more important, what antibodies are produced are less specific for the foreign antigen than in the younger animal. The result is that the antibodies cross-react with the animal's own cellular proteins; an autoimmune process is established. But the reaction of antibody with tissues of the host animal causes damage and loss of cells, as occurs with aging.

It has been suggested that the same disturbances in the genetic material described earlier which can result in faulty protein synthesis causes the production of nonspecific antibodies which cross-react and destroy host cells. There is also a decreased ability of the immune lymphocytes of old animals to proliferate in response to an antigenic challenge.

Our understanding at the present time of the aging process seems to indicate a relationship to the accumulation of mutational damage within the genetic mechanism of somatic cells. This leads to synthesis of defective proteins. Some of these proteins are essential enzymes within the cells, the loss of which will result in cell death. Other defective proteins may be antigenic and thus stimulate an immune response against the changed cell, while still other defective proteins may be antibodies with impaired specificity which cross-react with normal cell constituents, damaging or killing cells through an autoimmune process. It is thus unlikely that aging is due to a single cause but to the sum of many causes.

ORGAN AGING

The possibility has been considered repeatedly that some vital organ is programmed to undergo senescence. All the developmental changes which occur during embryonic life and during growth to the adult animal are genetically determined. The information for these changes exists in the DNA when the complement from the sperm joins that in the ovum at the moment of fertilization. Later events in life are also genetically determined. The failure of the ovaries in the female at the time of the menopause is such an instance of programmed death occurring at a time when other organs of the body are still highly viable. Perhaps some other organ more vital to the life of the individual than the ovaries is similarly programmed for extinction and determines the limit of life of the individual.

In the human female failure of function of the ovaries at menopause is accompanied by a large increase in the blood in the concentration of the follicle stimulating hormone (FSH) of the pituitary gland. Since ovarian function is dependent on this hormone, and since a similar increase in concentration accompanies surgical extirpation of the ovaries in the younger premenopausal female, it is generally regarded that the menopause in the human represents primary ovarian failure. This is an example of so-called "end-organ failure." Estrogen, the female hormone secreted by the ovary, suppresses the production of FSH by the pituitary. Only with ovarian failure and lack of estrogen is this inhibitory restraint released, permitting increased production of FSH by the pituitary. In the rat it has been claimed that transplantation of an inactive ovary from an elderly female to a young female will result in a resumption of activity by the elderly ovary. This would suggest that, in the rat, it is failure of trophic factors from pituitary or elsewhere which results in cessation of ovarian function rather than primary failure of the ovary, as in the human.

Observations such as these and the known regulatory role of hormones in promoting development and differentiation have led some investigators to study the endocrine system as a possible prime mover in the aging process. In addition to changes in the pituitary and sex glands other endocrine glands have been found to change their pattern of function with age. Thus the adrenal cortex has been shown to produce a relative excess of hormones which stimulate a breakdown of tissue in the elderly. Such a hormonal imbalance would be expected to facilitate a corresponding imbalance in the rate of protein synthesis and break down in favor of the latter. Loss of body protein is a characteristic of the aging process, as has been discussed. However, whether the hormonal changes are the cause of aging or simply the consequence of the aging process affecting the endocrine glands, is at present not known.

In addition to the endocrine system the other major integrator is the central nervous system. In fact, as knowledge of the regulation of function of various endocrine glands increases, the facts frequently lead us to lower portions of the brain which control several endocrine activities. Various releasing factors are now being discovered in the brain which then act upon the pituitary gland to secrete its trophic hormones. These regulatory activities in lower parts of the brain are undoubtedly connected with higher or cortical parts of the brain. The brain may thus influence growth and development of the body through the endocrine system or through direct connection via nerves with all parts of the body. We often hear the statement made in reference to someone who has suffered a particularly traumatic experience, "How much he has aged lately!" Where the experience has been a psychic one it is presumably the brain which has been responsible for the hastened pace of aging. It is significant in this regard that deterioration of mental faculties by psychological testing has been reported to be an earlier and more sensitive prognosticator of impending death than any findings on physical examination. As with the endocrine system it is not possible to state at present in regard to the brain and aging which is cause and which is effect.

It has often been pointed out that life is an improbable event. Matter in our universe gradually but inexorably moves toward a state of increased randomness with molecules moving in disorganized disarray as entropy increases. The Second Law of Thermodynamics is, of course, the statement of this tendency of matter to achieve maximal disorder. Living organisms, by contrast, depend for their existence on highly organized arrangements of matter; they live on "negative entropy," seeming to defy the natural command for confusion ever to increase. The molecules within the genes which contain the genetic information are among the most highly structured and ordered constituents of living systems. Thus information is an improbable occurrence, just as is life. The Second Law applied to information, which is order, predicts the increase in misinformation, "noise," or garbling of information which is expressed in living matter as senescence and ultimate death. It is not surprising that aging is an expected natural process and that it results from mistakes or randomness developing within the genetic information of cells and in the translation of this misinformation into the synthetic reactions on which life depends. It is remarkable that the flimsy strands of DNA can preserve the genetic message for as long as does occur in spite of all the environmental factors operating to increase randomness even in these molecules. The specific manifestations of this increasing misinformation in the gene will undoubtedly reveal themselves in many disorders of synthesis, structure, and function of cellular components, until the cell itself is no longer viable. It is thus unlikely that aging is due to a single cause but rather to the sum of many causes affecting the genetic apparatus and its expression in somatic cells. Fortunately, the genetic material in our germ cells (ova and sperm) largely escapes this random disorganization or its consequences and thereby preserves species immortality.

The aim of gerontologists is to learn the details by which genetic information becomes garbled and how the garbled messages lead to synthesis of cellular constituents which no longer can function in the harmonious state known as "life." Only through understanding of the specific molecular disorders that accrue with time will ability potentially to modify or prevent these disorders occur.

Much more research is needed before the necessary details will be understood. Until better understanding of the aging process itself is achieved there is little likelihood, it seems to me, that the maximum life span can be extended for man. Many different factors of the environment, of metabolism, and of the genes will most probably be found to be involved.

12

SOCIAL CONSEQUENCES OF AN EXTENDED LIFE SPAN

Young men think old men are fools;
But old men know young men are fools.
George Chapman (1557–1634), *All Fools,* Act V, Scene 1

One cannot discuss the possibility of either extending the human life span or increasing the proportion of elderly individuals in our population without serious thought to the potential social, economic, and political consequences. Volumes could and have been written on the subject, and only a brief commentary will be included here. But to consider extending the life span without thinking and planning for the possible consequence to our crowded world would be immoral, to say the least.

According to the 1970 census there were 20,066,000 persons in the United States who were sixty-five or older. This constitutes 9.3 percent of our population. In some states, the local average exceeds the national average by a considerable margin—e.g., Florida has 14.6 percent of its population sixty-five years of age or older. This trend toward an increasing percentage of the population in the older age group is prevalent throughout the industrialized world.

At the Ninth International Congress of Gerontology in Kiev in 1972, Professor M. Vacek of Czechoslovakia discussed the increase in mean age and the rising proportion of old people in the population. He pointed out that the rise in the proportion of people over sixty-five toward fifteen percent in the populations of stable industrial countries was attributable to a falling birth rate. When at the conclusion of his talk, someone in the audience timidly asked if the great achievements of modern medicine had played a role in the rise in mean age, he responded that indeed they had, but that the simultaneous deterioration of the environment had canceled out any positive effect from medicine.

Mere length of life, however, is not the issue on which this book is focused. Most would agree that the quality of life, rather than its duration, should be the prime concern. The active life so warmly espoused by Theodore Roosevelt has been the American model. If one can extend the period of productive activity as did Verdi and Churchill, so much the better. But even with an increased proportion of vigorous active oldsters, new problems will arise, and if in time the actual biological limits of life can be pushed back significantly the issues confronting society will be enormous.

It is a natural tendency to think in very personal terms regarding the possibility of extending the life span. I am sure that Ponce de León thought only about the advantages and pleasures for himself of finding the Fountain of Youth.

What advantages might there be to prolonging life, assuming that mental and physical abilities were preserved? My father used to look up from his books while my brothers and I struggled with our school homework and remark, "Unfortunately you must relearn everything I learned. My knowledge I cannot give you; it goes with me." We are destined each to start with a clean slate. This may have advantages but a significant portion of our life span is devoted to this learning process before we return this investment to society. As science and technology become more sophisticated this portion of the life span has increased. Surgical and medical specialists may not complete their formal training until the age of thirty or thirty-two. Only then are they certified to practice independently. Clearly an extension of their active professional life beyond ages sixty-five to seventy would yield a greater return to society for the costly investment in time and resources made during the long period of education and training. Medicine may represent an extreme example of prolonged formal training, but the same principle applies to many other occupations in which experience makes a difference. For lawyers, engineers, businessmen, teachers, judges, nurses, craftsmen, writers, executives, and many others in our culture, experience enriches their performance or creativity. If the period during which their skills were enhanced by experience could be extended without the adverse effects of aging restricting this gain, prolongation of the active, functional life span would benefit society.

Certainly a society dominated by its older citizens will be a conservative one, resistant to change. It is therefore likely to be more stable. These qualities may only be social virtues if the form of the society is worth maintaining. It seems to me that a social order merits preservation only if it permits opportunity for full expression of the individual's abilities in directions which don't compromise the welfare of others. If a society dominated by older citizens is compatible with this criterion, then stability may be worthwhile. Because of changes in the aging brain, as described earlier, decreased ability to adapt psychologically to new situations leads to preoccupation with the familiar. This psychological conservatism—resistance to change—together with his more established position in society tends to make the older citizen support the status quo, which in turn protects his privileged position. This is generally accomplished by the manipulation of wealth, which he has had a longer time to acquire than the young.

With an extension of the vigorous active life span we may anticipate that the development of fixed thought and behavior patterns will also be delayed. In fact, the sprightly elderly are often characterized by the resilience of their minds. This is no coincidence. Jarvik, Kallman, and associates had demonstrated a possible association between intellectual performance and survival in their longitudinal study of aging twins. They found that surviving twins had attained higher scores on a battery of psychomotor tests than did the deceased. It wasn't that the survivors were initially brighter than the deceased; the results showed that the performance of the survivors on the psychological tests decreased more slowly. Such psychological changes, they found, may precede evident physiological deterioration and thus serve as prognosticators of the probability of survival. By contrast, general age-related decline on tasks involving fast motor coordination was not correlated with survival. For the point of the present discussion such information encourages me to expect that a prolonged, physically healthy life will be associated with a preservation of mental adaptability and resiliency. Thus, fears that extension of the life span must lead to an increased population of elders rigidified in their thinking and behavior patterns can be allayed.

It has been suggested that many of the antisocial characteristics exhibited by members of today's societies—greed, avarice, wastefulness, prejudices—are fostered by the shortness of our present life span, and that with a longer time to establish our position we could afford to be less selfish and grasping, it is argued. We would see our children grow to adulthood quite capable of providing for themselves, so there would be no need presumably to amass fortunes for the security of offspring. With less individual competitiveness there might be a decrease in nationalism and in the friction between countries based on economic competition. Wars would disappear and wasteful destruction of the environment would cease. Utopia would result simply from an extension of the human life span, so the daydream goes.

Unfortunately there is no certainty that a longer life span would not simply permit a more prolonged period for man to exercise all his antisocial capabilities. If such were to be the case, better that the life span be shortened! However, it is probably not justified to take either an extremely optimistic or pessimistic view in this matter.

Over many thousands of years of evolution man has developed in a hostile world in which those who survived and procreated were those whose qualities of self-sufficiency and -preservation were most highly developed. Self-interest, aggression, independence, and a large measure of selfishness were necessary traits for survival. In a world that has become increasingly interdependent, in which societal and economic cooperation can provide the individual with many benefits, the old atavistic individual values may actually hinder individual welfare. Man in our present industrialized nations has been singularly unsuccessful to date in subjugating personal self-interest in the interests of the cooperation which is needed in our small interdependent world. Adherence to characteristics that served the individual so well in a primitive world can hardly be in the best long-range interests of mankind at a time when means of mass human destruction are at hand and rape of the environment, of precious, irreplaceable natural beauty and resources, occurs at the whim of economic self-interest. It is our inability to live together that constitutes the major threat to the future. The fruits of science and technology are all too often perverted into means of destruction rather than to the benefit of all. We need to learn more realistic ways to coexist with one another and with our precious world. Perhaps a longer life span would provide the time necessary for us to subdue selfish individual characteristics and replace them with socially constructive patterns of behavior. Perhaps this view requires acquisition of a public wisdom for which there is no precedent in history—and even a longer life will not accomplish this.

I have no doubt strayed far beyond the limits of the license permitted to a physician commenting on health and longevity. But individual health and longevity is not likely if it is nurtured in a schizophrenic society bent on its self-destruction. The duty of the physician is to the health of the individual, but that cannot flourish optimally except in a healthy society. The physician perhaps more than others can thus not logically shirk his social obligations.

To return to more mundane aspects of increasing the human life span, the potential medical costs must be examined. Today, with ten percent of our population over the age of sixty-five, this segment consumed a quarter of the expenditure for health care in the United States. Since the total expenditure amounted to $94 billion in 1973, the medical costs of an aging population are not trivial. One would hope that any extension of the active life span would be terminated by a short illness after additional years of low morbidity. There is no assurance, however, that such will be the case. If fact, if the present killers—heart attacks, strokes, and cancer—are eradicated or their occurrence postponed on the average by several decades, it is possible that arthritis and other disabling or debilitating ailments might "increase" to curse the added years. The responsibility to assure that years added to our life span are years of vigorous health is a major one that anyone who works in this area must accept. That is why I am so convinced that the route of primary prevention which must start with concern and care for health at an early age is the only way a worthwhile extension of the lifespan can be attained.

How will a role be created for the old people which can replace the central position they held in the extended family group in an agrarian economy? The importance of a socially useful role for the elderly has been emphasized—and, I believe, cannot be overemphasized. The trend today seems to be to sequester our elders in housing projects for the elderly or even villages for the golden years. I see no way that our modern economy can absorb the increasing number of elderly citizens back into the labor force or into previously held important managerial or professional activities.

A panel of the World Health Organization has recently heard expert opinion state that older people in the poorer countries are often better off than are old people in the more affluent nations. The older people in these poorer lands, the experts say, still enjoy status because of their age, something lost in the industrialized nations. Furthermore, their care is primarily a matter of family responsibility. By contrast, in the industrialized advanced countries, the aged were more often fully or partly dependent on the state for support, the WHO study shows. The study further notes that the compulsory retirement that prevails today in advanced countries brings with it loss of status, reduction of social contacts and decrease in income. The aged, it is stressed, would be physically and mentally better off and would enjoy a higher standing in society if their productive activities were maintained at an optimal level in relation to their capacity.

Attempts to create or preserve jobs by retarding efficiency of production through suppressing automation or application of new technology seem retrogressive to me. But ways will have to be found to let everyone share in the benefits of these efficiencies; the economy should have as its function service to people's needs rather than the reverse roles. Assignment to hard physical employment for life, if no longer essential for survival, seems a high cost to pay for a long life. That such labor was a necessity in the relatively primitive cultures I visited points up the need for continued physical activity and psychological involvement in society—but does not mean that both can be achieved only through onerous labor. Surely we can all find enjoyable pursuits to fill our leisure hours with purpose if we consciously encourage development of human service and avocations early in our lives. Habits of regular physical exercise can also be cultivated.

It seems, therefore, that interests—creative and service activities— cultivated in earlier years will have to provide the raison d'être and the day-to-day satisfactions. Where proximity permits frequent contacts with family, certainly the grandparents will benefit, as will the grandchildren. Any activity with family or community which gives a sense of purpose and usefulness will sustain the elderly. It seems to me that this aspect of providing the needed psychological support will be the factor most difficult to achieve. How much are we willing and able to change our living patterns and social customs to accommodate the elderly? Even the realization that all too soon we will be they hardly seems to stem the trends which now ostracize the elderly.

Research in the psychological needs of the elderly is very much needed. I have been assuming that a need to be useful in the social and economic life of the family or community exists as almost a fundamental requirement. It is true that agrarian societies I visited provided for this need. Perhaps there are other ways to motivate the desire to live and some of these ways could be provided by our society without the inconvenience and stress of absorbing the elderly back into the mainstream of our economic life. I suspect that interests and skills which could be taught and fostered in our educational system might provide the needed, sustaining gratifications. It is this continuation of enjoyment and gratification that the elderly need. "We [and the elderly] do not live by bread alone!"

How would we support an increased proportion of elderly citizens who were no longer contributing gainfully to the economy? Clearly our social security and old-age pension system would have to be bolstered. Earnings generated during a relatively shortened productive portion of the life span would have to be stretched to afford economic security in old age. Although private initiative through savings and investments might suffice for some, it has become the expectation that government will assume a large responsibility in supporting the elderly. This should be efficiently accomplished through support of socially useful activities rather than by means of a direct dole.

Even with the old people remaining vigorous and active, their contributions to the economy are not likely to be required to sustain a large Gross National Product. The situation I witnessed in Abkhasia is not likely to be repeated here. There, in the village of Kutol, I talked to Khfaf Lasuria, who is some 130 years old. She lives on a collective farm and had been gainfully employed until two years prior to my visit. Still sprightly and enjoying herself she has retired and has received a pension from the government only for the past two years! Our economy doesn't need such devoted and prolonged individual support. But it will be complicated and require the cooperation and foresight of wage earners and business to cooperate with government to create an effective alternative to Khfaf Lasuria's method of supporting herself by her own labors for the first 128 years of her life.

A moral question must yet be answered. Overpopulation with attendent malnutrition, starvation, poverty, and misery is today a major problem. The myth that food supplies can keep abreast of human fecundity and even that available energy supplies were unlimited and inexhaustible has been exploded by recent events. Not only gross malnutrition, but starvation and death threaten large population groups in Asia and Africa today. At the same time, the industrialized nations are consuming resources and despoiling our natural environment at an unprecedented rate. What will happen if we add to this situation the burden of providing the needs of an increasing population of elders?

The only tenable accommodation would be to reduce births and hold down the population in this manner. Families will need to be smaller if we are to keep in balance with available resources. It is, of course, a personal judgment made with minimal facts as to how crowded we can become without suffering the consequences. To me it seems that the quality of life will suffer from too many people long before we have crowded the last person onto our planet whom we can still feed, clothe, and house. The human species has had unprecedented biologic success in expanding its numbers. But this very biologic success stands now as the greatest threat to the survival of our species. We have done little yet to control population growth, depending with blind faith on science and technology to delay the day of reckoning when the rate of consumption can no longer be matched by the rate of production for our needs. A general willingness to slow the rate of consumption by lowering the standard of living, especially in the more advanced societies which have the highest per capita consumption rate, will delay but probably not prevent the crisis. If our numbers continue to increase it will likely be the food supply that becomes the limiting factor in survival, but problems of waste disposal may be equally serious. Before that day arrives the value of human life will have cheapened. Individuals and finally nations will fight for available supplies. With present means of destruction, such a situation may lead to destruction of civilization and perhaps even of our species. Spiders have a tolerance to radioactive irradiation which is much greater than ours; perhaps the future will belong to them!

Thus it seems to me we must deal urgently with the population problem. Since population growth is geometric—has the nature of a chain reaction—it becomes increasingly difficult to slow down the absolute growth the larger the population base.

How can I justify consciously extending the average life span against the backdrop of gloom that has just been described? I believe that each individual born should have an opportunity to grow up healthy, be educated, be gainfully employed—in one way or another to make a positive contribution to the needs of society and have his fair share of the prosperity to which he has contributed. If this opportunity is in jeopardy because of too many mouths to feed, then control measures—voluntary, one hopes—are needed. I feel that, if this opportunity is a commitment of society to the individual, then it must be kept throughout the life of the individual. If the life span can be extended with vigorous, enjoyable, active years, then the population control should be on the birth rate. The obligation must be to the living not to the unborn who potentially are almost limitless in numbers. If we improve the quality of life for the present living, those born later will share the benefit.

Clearly our values, our life style, and a good deal of our

thinking will need to change if conditions are to be created in which a long, vigorous, healthy life is socially desirable. But, since I believe that the same conditions are necessary for all to have a full life regardless of its length, it seems never too soon to create the conditions.

DO'S AND DON'TS

The art of living consists of dying young—but as late as possible!

Anonymous

It must be evident by now that current thinking would lead to the conclusion that longevity is a multifactorial condition. When these several factors occur simultaneously in favorable combination, long life is attained. It has ever been the hope of man that some single factor, potion, or pill will be discovered which will alone assure good health and a long happy life. This hope has spawned many, many fads and frauds throughout the ages. Today, if one surveys the scene, there is little evidence that we are significantly less gullible than our forebears.

A search for a magic spring whose waters would confer eternal youth on its drinker inspired Ponce de León inadvertently to discover Florida. Most fads involve either frank magic or pseudo-science. Extracts of various herbs, mandrake root, partridge brains, salep (a powder from the tubers of orchids), birds'-nest soup—all are still utilized for their presumed magical powers. In Vilcabamba we heard repeatedly from the elderly males that they attributed their long lives to their custom of bathing in the blood of animals freshly killed in the hunt. This explanation will strike any reader who has persisted with me this far as highly improbable. And yet we all read or hear claims for this vitamin preparation, that hormone injection, colonic irrigations, gland treatments, mineral waters, bee-collected pollen, diet fads, and many other of "nature's complete revitalizing treatments" with a quickening of interest. After all, what is there to lose? Why not play it safe just in case there is something to the unsubstantiated claims? After all, the claims sound plausible—and often more so than many of the hunches upon which so many of our actions or decisions are based.

For the more educated and affluent clientele there are more sophisticated treatments to entice, and there seems never to be a shortage of patients, including the famous and the wealthy. Dr. Ana Aslan of Bucharest developed a product, Gerovital, twenty years ago which is largely the standard local anesthetic agent, procaine or novocaine. Dr. Aslan claims her product is effective against arthritis, arteriosclerosis, and the general infirmities of old age. She has treated Nikita Khrushchev, who was enthusiastic over the results, as well as Sukarno, Ho Chi Minh, and some Western notables. There has been interest among respected gerontologists in this country to obtain permission from our Food and Drug Administration to perform a controlled trial of Gerovital. Interestingly, Aslan claims that American procaine lacks the curative and revitalizing action of the Rumanian compound; she states that only her product is effective.

Another recent and very lucrative fad is cell or organ therapy. This form of quackery had an auspicious start. It was the highly respected French physician and physiologist, Dr. Charles Edouard Brown-Sequard, who started it and was the first subject. He had a distinguished career as a physiologist and neurologist in France, England, and the United States, including an appointment as professor of physiology and pathology of the nervous system at Harvard and the chair of experimental pathology at the Faculty of Medicine in Paris. Later he succeeded the great physiologist Claude Bernard at the Collège de France. He is generally credited with being a founder of modern endocrinology. His credentials were impeccable, and he created no little excitement when in 1889, at the age of seventy-two, he injected himself with an extract prepared from animal testicles and claimed that it made a new man of him. Brown-Sequard told a distinguished academic audience in Paris that after three injections he had turned the clock back thirty years. "Today I was able to pay a visit to the young Madame Brown-Sequard," he concluded, incontrovertible testimony to the success of his new treatment. This success launched a busy practice injecting thousands who came to be similarly revitalized with the liquid extracted from pulverized bulls' testicles. Brown-Sequard, however, soon found himself in difficulties with his professional colleagues.

The idea that Brown-Sequard had has reappeared in modified form. Dr. Serge Voronoff, also working in France, made himself famous by implanting pieces of chimpanzee testicles in male patients. Many flocked to Paris to receive his monkey-gland treatments. Whereas Brown-Sequard may have been providing his patients with some testosterone, the major male sex hormone, with the injections he gave, transplanted foreign tissue is rapidly rejected by the host, and Voronoff's patients could have received very little even of testosterone from this treatment.

In 1920 Dr. Paul Niehans took up the transplantation of endocrine glands and had some success in animal experiments.

In the 1930s he apparently found that the same procedures performed in humans were much more lucrative. His claim was that cells taken from animal organs would revitalize by some mysterious means the corresponding organ in patients injected with cells. The large and very busy cell therapy business which he established in his exclusive private clinic, La Prani, in Switzerland, is still thriving financially; and the practice is spreading elsewhere, since there seem to be many of the world's affluent seeking treatment. Fortunately in the United States we are protected by strict Food and Drug Administration regulations from such practices. But even in England such treatments are conducted openly and profitably. Niehans, who throughout a long career was always vague as to the mechanism by which cell therapy benefited his patients, was always positive about its effectiveness. He recommended heart cells for damaged hearts; placenta cells for exhaustion after childbirth, for hypertension, and for angina; and injections of hypothalamus cells for "sexual neurasthenia." Cells for these injections were supplied fresh largely from ewe's fetuses in a private abattoir in his clinic. Among his patients allegedly were King George VI and Pope Pius XII.

Today a practitioner of cell therapy can obtain fresh-frozen, vacuum-packed cells ready to be injected—and the practice is spreading. Often patients are quite willing to offer testimony to such treatments. One quite extravagant claim made for cell-therapy appeared in a recent exposé of the practice by Paul Ferris in the New York Times. The patient, age sixty-three, alleged that two years following cell therapy he was relieved of arthritic pains from which he had suffered for the preceding fifteen years despite trying all the orthodox treatments. He was the recipient of serum from thyroid, pituitary, thymus, adrenal, testes, heart, arteries, liver, spleen, kidney, lung, skin, intestines, and the reticuloendothelial system during his course of cell therapy. As a bonus the patient found his sex life markedly improved: "When I was younger," he stated, "I could have three or four orgasms with the same erection. For the past ten or eleven years, I've not been able to do that—until after my first treatment. Now I can manage multiple orgasms once or twice a month, which isn't bad at sixty-three." Such claims are irresistible to enough affluent persons to perpetuate the treatments.

Orthodox medicine takes a very skeptical attitude toward such treatments. It is not the veracity or sincerity of the proponents which is always in question, nor is it the possibility that the motivation of the therapist is purely monetary. It is the fact that, when forms of therapy are not subjected to rigorously controlled study, bias may so affect the results that the truth of whether or not actual physical benefit results from the treatment may never be known. Since there is almost always some risk involved in the taking of any medications, as well as costs, it is important that efficacy of the therapy be established. The claims for success of such treatments as we have been discussing are always anecdotal, and whether the patient's illness would have spontaneously ameliorated or whether a placebo given with the same conviction and assurance would have proven to be equally successful, cannot be judged. It is a controlled trial that orthodox medicine demands—though, of course, it hastens acceptance if a rational explanation for a beneficial effect according to known principles of physiology or biochemistry is available. But there is so much that we don't yet know that it is the proof of beneficial effect even more than the understanding of the effect that is demanded. Physicians prescribe adrenal hormones for rheumatoid arthritis, vasculitis, endotoxic shock, ulcerative colitis, and other conditions in which the mechanism for the apparent beneficial action is not yet understood. In fact, there are generally so many variable factors present in any diseased state that it requires relatively little ingenuity to produce a plausible explanation for an effect; to prove the correctness of the explanation, however, is often a very much more difficult matter. But medicine will accept the controlled trial as evidence for incorporating the agent into its therapeutic armamentarium.

The concept of the controlled trial is very simple, indeed. One divides patients into two groups randomly so that no selection occurs in the assignment into the control and the experimental group. Alternatively patients may be matched in the two groups for age, sex, severity of illness, and other factors which might serve to modify the effects of therapy. Then the experimental group is given the treatment to be tested, while the control group is kept on conventional therapy or given a placebo in place of the treatment. In some test designs, each subject may serve as his own control; or after a time the control and experimental groups may be switched, so that the former control group is given the treatment under question and the former treatment group serves as control. A variety of experimental designs and numbers of patients included may be utilized according to the statistical requirements of the study. Criteria for judging success of therapy are stated beforehand: usually some objective finding, such as abatement of fever, change in blood counts or in blood chemistry tests, or alteration in the electrocardiogram, is picked, so that end points are readily recognizable and not subject to observer bias. Sometimes a subjective relief of pain or other symptom is the only effect of treatment, and the patient's subjective impression becomes the end point. In this situation alternations of treatment and placebo without patient or therapist knowing which the patient is actually receiving (the so-called "double-blind study") may be necessary in order to validate an effect. Therapist bias, as much as patient bias, may be an important factor in the results if not also rigorously controlled.

Clearly, the rigorous testing of any new therapeutic measure, though simple in principle, may become very costly and difficult. It may require great skill and perseverance on the part of the clinical investigator. When such questions as an effect on the life span of a given treatment are asked, the experimental and control groups may have to be observed over many years. This is why knowledge in this field is so difficult to come by. This is why the field is so fertile for the charlatan. A controlled study is generally the last thing he is interested in, and without such a study it is often impossible for the legitimate practitioner to swear that there can be no value to the charlatan's treatments. He may only counter the claims as not being rigorously proven. This often leaves the medical profession looking very reactionary and unwilling to accept new treatments. But the medical profession has learned from long and often painful experience that, no matter how sensational the claims are for a new treatment, it must be subjected to a control trial for ultimate proof. Of course, if the new treatment is as effective as penicillin in the treatment of pneumonia caused by the pneumococcus, then the comparison is easily performed and the number of patients involved in such tests need only be few. However, if the effectiveness of the new treatment at best is only marginal, the number of patients involved may need to be very large.

The successful quack is very clever. He knows the power of suggestion. He knows that most complaints are functional—that is, have their basis in emotional tensions, insecurities, anxieties, nervousness, personal conflicts, rather than in demonstrable organic pathology. When the patient comes seeking treatment and is willing to pay a high price for it, there is little more that the quack need do but give the injection (it should be a little painful) and collect the fee (large enough also to be painful). The patient will do the rest. Not to improve requires admission by the patient to himself that he has been gullible and swindled because of his foolishness—an admission that most of us will try very hard to avoid. The quack has everything in his favor, and, if the effects of the treatments are to prolong the life span of the subject, many years are likely to pass before the success or failure can be judged. The quack can practice his fraud with impunity if he uses only a little common sense and restricts his trade to relatively healthy individuals. It must have been such considerations which led Benjamin Franklin to state, "Quacks are the greatest liars in the world—except their patients."

Many fads and fashions for promoting longevity have come and gone—many more undoubtedly will appear. H. P. von Hahn has aptly stated the responsible viewpoint: "I believe that our present understanding of the changes occurring in cells and tissues when they age shows that these changes are in general permanent and irreversible. An effective therapy of aging can therefore only be a preventive therapy. Rejuvenation is something we must leave to mythology." What can be said now to guide the reader intelligently toward a longer, healthier life?

From his study of ancestry of long-lived individuals R. Pearl advised aspirants to a long life to choose parents who themselves attained an old age. Genetic factors indeed are important, but unfortunately few of us have the opportunity to pick our parents. Thus it is encouraging that environmental factors are also of great importance. L. I. Dublin in his study of life insurance data found that offspring of long lived parents have a mean life expectancy at age twenty which does not exceed that of offspring of parents who were short lived by more than three years. This was the maximum advantage conferred by a favorable heredity according to his analysis. By contrast the extension of the life expectancy at birth from forty-eight years in 1900 to seventy years in 1969 was accomplished entirely by improving environmental determinants—it is true that the major improvement was the reduction in infant mortality.

In an article entitled, "Prospects for further increase in average longevity," B. Woodhall and S. Jablon have estimated from 1950 census figures the effect of eradicating major illnesses on average life expectancy. If cancer were no longer a cause of death, another two years for males and 2.6 years for females would be added to the average life expectancy at birth. If cardio-vascular diseases (chiefly coronary heart disease and strokes) were deleted, the gain would be ten years for both sexes. Elimination of infections and parasitic diseases would add only 1.1 years for males and 0.9 years for females. This indicates that major progress in this area in the past fifty years leaves the possibility for only modest further statistical, as opposed to individual, gain in the United States. Prevention of accidents, suicides, and homicides would increase life expectancy for white males by 2.2 years. These are all conditions in which environmental factors play a large causative role. Eradication of the cardiovascular diseases alone would produce perhaps a nine percent relative increase in the proportion of the population over the age of sixty-five.

I have referred in detail previously to nutrition, physical activity, and psychological factors as important environmental determinants of health and longevity. Here these and other controllable influences will be briefly mentioned.

In the United States today our national eating habits are costly, wasteful, and unhealthy. It is true that the decrease in general malnutrition has improved our resistance to infections and caused us to grow taller. But a good thing can be carried too far and today we are an overfed nation. From what I saw on my travels and from medical experience I would advise a caloric intake considerably below the minimum daily allowances recommended by the National Academy of Sciences and the National Research Council. With our increasingly sedentary life, the caloric requirements probably rarely exceed 2500 calories for males at any time in life or 2000 calories per day for females. Some thirty calories per kilogram *lean body weight* per day will generally suffice. There will be great variations in individual needs and body weight is the best indication of caloric adequacy provided that an optimal lean body weight is chosen as the norm. Weight should not increase with age, and for most persons their weight at the time that full body growth has been attained, at ages eighteen to twenty, generally should be kept with expectation of gradual decline after sixty. The metabolic rate for old people is the same as for younger adults on a cell for cell basis. However, both the number of cells and activity decrease with age, and hence so do caloric needs.

It should be remembered that actual caloric undernutrition (as compared with intake as desired) during the period of development remains the most reliable means of extending the life span in the experimental animal. On such caloric-restricted, but otherwise adequate diets, experimental animals are also protected from most illnesses. Such studies, for obvious reasons, cannot be conscientiously performed on humans; yet they suggest that after the first year or two, when the brain has acquired its full complement of cells, we would do well not to overfeed our infants and children. In adult individuals of average body weight J. Hirsch and associates estimated the total number of fat cells to average 27 times 10^9. They found that the normal growth and development of the fat tissue comes about by cellular multiplication rather than enlargement. The number of fat cells increases into late adolescence or early adult life. It appears that once the adult number of cells is achieved, weight reduction occurs by a decrease in fat content of each cell but not by a decrease in the number of fat cells; they remain ever present and ever ready to be restuffed. In extremely obese subjects they found the size of individual fat cells to be essentially the same as in the normal. The striking finding was an increase in the total number of fat cells, which may be two to five times normal. Overfeeding during the early years of life, when fat cells are still multiplying, may stimulate their increased numbers.

In referring to the costly and wasteful nature of our diets I refer primarily to our intake of protein. For males fifteen to fifty-five years of age, this exceeds 100 grams daily; for females, the figure exceeds 70 grams daily for the same age interval. Thirty grams of protein of high nutritive value—i.e., with adequate content of essential amino acids, as in milk proteins and meat—will sustain body protein stores if the diet contains adequate additional calories from carbohydrates and fats. Thus 60 grams of protein should provide an adequate margin of safety for normal adults. The requirements do not seem to change with old age.

There is little evidence that the high protein intake we ingest is directly injurious to health if normal kidney function is present to excrete the toxic waste products of protein metabolism. But milk and meat proteins generally come associated with high fat and cholesterol intake and the concomitant high intake of these food substances is undesirable. One should also remember that in rough figures the grazing land required to produce one pound of meat if utilized for agriculture would provide the equivalent of sixteen times as many calories in grains, legumes, and vegetables. Thus, in a hungry world, meat production is costly in arable land—as well as costly to the consumer.

The role of fats in the development or protection of athero-sclerosis has been discussed in detail. Saturated animal fats, i.e., meat fats and butterfat, are associated with high cholesterol and blood lipid levels and atherosclerosis. Although evidence for a causal relationship is not absolutely compelling, the association seems to me a strong one—sufficiently convincing that it deserves a reduction in these sources of fat in our diets and their replacement by polyunsaturated fats which derive largely from vegetable sources. Furthermore, the absolute level of fat in our diets, which may exceed 120 grams per day for males in the age range of fifteen to thirty-four years, should be reduced. In addition to a potential contribution to atherosclerosis, the extra calories simply are not needed by most of us. Reducing meat and dairy products in our diets in favor of vegetable foods will accomplish both goals. Poultry and fish are preferable to red meats. Milk without its butterfat remains an excellent source of high quality protein and fortunately is available and inexpensive as fat free milk solids.

Highly refined sugars and carbohydrates are also unfortunate intruders into our modern menus—in fact, so ubiquitous as to be taken for granted as major staples. As a nation we now ingest 120 pounds of sucrose-purified common sugar—per person per year. Refined carbohydrates have also been blamed for high blood neutral fat and cholesterol levels and for an increased incidence of heart attacks. The process of refining strips the grain and flour of all its vitamins and minerals. Thus sucrose and white flour should be avoided in favor of whole grain and unrefined carbohy-drates. We have already mentioned the value of the fiber and bran associated with unrefined carbohydrates and grains in preventing constipation and the hypothesis that a more rapid transit time through the colon may reduce the occurrence of cancer of the colon.

The deleterious, caries-inducing effect of high sucrose feedings on dentition has been long recognized. An interesting recent hypothesis attributes obesity and excessive caloric intake to the ingestion of purified carbohydrate. The idea is that, stripped of their fiber content, refined carbohydrates are rapidly absorbed, leaving the intestines empty and thus providing little satiety value. This encourages more frequent, larger feedings and obesity. Ingestion of unrefined carbohydrates with their fiber content fills the stomach with fewer calories, appeasing appetite without excessive caloric intake. Further, with an increase in the content of fiber within the small bowel there is actual interference with fat absorption so that some increased fat and hence calories appear in the stool. How significant this last effect of the fiber content of foods may be has not yet been established.

Much has been written and said regarding vitamin and mineral requirements. If the diet is diversified and contains fresh vegetables, both green and yellow, whole grain, and fresh fruits, then there should be no need for supplementary vitamins. But vitamin requirements may vary considerably from person to person and in the same person during ill health. Special circumstances, such as the state of dentition, may affect food consumption so as to produce imbalances. A physician's advice regarding diet should be sought under such circumstances.

The situation with respect to mineral requirements is even less clear. Discussions of nutrition generally include calcium, iron, and perhaps iodine but usually no other minerals. Many other elements are essential parts of important body constituents but almost nothing is known regarding nutritional requirements for them. Requirements for iron can be most precisely defined, since the number of circulating red blood cells is dependent on the adequacy of the iron stores in the body. An even more sensitive test for the adequacy of iron stores is the percent saturation with iron of the binding capacity of a special binding protein in plasma. Iodine needs are generally satisfied by the use of iodized salt, which has diminished the incidence of goiter due to iodine deficiency and essentially abolished cretinism in the United States. Iodine deficiency persists as an important health problem, however, in some parts of the world.

The requirements for calcium remain a topic for debate and study. There is no question that a growing child has definite requirements for calcium and phosphorus during the stage of bone growth and mineralization. The dietary requirements are related to the vitamin D levels since this vitamin is essential for the normal process of calcium absorption from the intestines. In the adult calcium is also needed, but in smaller amounts, to replace the bone calcium, which is in a continuous state of turnover (calcification and decalcification). The major problem is that of osteoporosis of aging. This is a gradual loss of mineral from the bones making up the axial skeleton which occurs all too commonly among our elderly. The cause of this atrophy of bone is not yet understood, but it is a major cause of disability and discomfort among the aged. It seems that simply increasing dietary calcium, even with additional vitamin D, has little if any beneficial affect on the osteoporosis. The apparent lack of osteoporosis among the elderly in the places I visited seems related to their continuous physical activity, which may thus be more important than dietary factors in preventing atrophy of bone.

Most important, good dietary habits should be established in early life. Animal experiments indicate that diet in the perinatal period (birth) may importantly influence longevity. Certainly what one eats during his first, second, third, fourth, and fifth decades may be as important as what he eats at age eighty or 100.

The internist is frequently asked about the effect of alcohol intake on health. Obviously when drunk in large amounts it is highly injurious to the liver, brain, and other organs. By reducing inhibitions it often leads to overeating when taken before meals; when taken without the food it can lead to severe malnutrition from vitamin and protein deficiency. In all three areas visited the old people partook of some alcoholic beverage, but usually in moderation. A recent study suggested that one cocktail a day may actually be conducive to decreased mortality from cardiovascular diseases. Whether individuals who consume a daily cocktail happen to be longer lived for other reasons isn't clear. Surely the benefit, if any, is not nutritional, but possibly is the relaxing and sociabilizing effect of small amounts of alcohol. A dictum of one of my colleagues points up a major difficulty with the control of alcholic consumption: "One drink is enough, two are too many, and three aren't nearly enough!" If you can't stop at one or two drinks it is best not to start at all.

I have discussed in some detail the importance of exercise to health. But the form of the exercise is important. "Brute" sports which require great strength have perhaps negative survival value. The mean age at death of football players in one report was fifty-seven years. Exercise should be regular, frequent, and continued throughout life. I tend to agree with the recent claims of a group called the American Medical Joggers Association that endurance exercises are most beneficial. They state that not speed or strength but endurance is what counts—and that "physical fitness means endurance." Long walks, jogging, cross-country skiing, swimming, rowing, and bicycle riding are the sports recommended. These are activities which can be paced so as not to be strenuous, and nearly anyone can participate provided that he starts modestly and increases activity gradually.

Anyone who is over forty starting a physical fitness program should have a medical examination including an electrocardiogram. Abnormalities on the electrocardiogram do not necessarily preclude a program of physical activity, but it should be undertaken with close medical supervision. There is ample evidence today that physical exercise is an important aspect of rehabilitation for those who have already experienced a heart attack. The program of exercises should be a graded one under careful medical supervision. For those who receive a clean bill of health a regular program of exercise should be instituted. The form of exercise may include any of those listed. It should be done regularly, preferably at least three times weekly. The exercise should be continued to the point of stressing the heart and lungs moderately, that is, until shortness of breath and an increase in heart rate to at least 120 but not more than 140 beats per minute occur. Endurance, not speed, is the goal, and this will entail gradually increasing the distance involved as the heart and lungs improve their performance. For me, jogging has been effective and economical of time. The cost of a good pair of running shoes has been my only investment for a million dollars' worth of well-being. My initial apprehensions over the ludicrous figure I must present were rapidly laid to rest when I found that even the neighborhood dogs totally ignored me. Thirty minutes at least three or more times a week devoted to such exercise will be beneficial.

In all three countries visited I found the old people participating in the social and economic life of community and family. The need seems to be for a role which sustains the self-esteem of the individual. No one can feel useless, unwanted, and redundant and survive for long. We each need to develop hobbies and interests which will provide for us a useful, enjoyable role compatible with our perception of ourselves and which sustain our status within our peer group. As leisure time increases we must develop such activities for our early as well as our late years. Society and government will have to yield considerably to help meet these psychological needs of the elderly in a supportive manner. A long life is worth living only if there is something worth living for.

I could go on to interdict smoking, drugs, environmental pollution, and all the many things today that we do individually or socially to create disease and shorten our life span, but these you can enumerate as well as I. The problem is why so many of us persist in activities which we know to be injurious to health. This is an individual matter which must be thought through and answered by each of us.

In this writing I have divulged no secrets nor provided any surprises—there just aren't any yet. But, if I can offer you no guaranteed formula of my own of how to attain a long vigorous healthy life, let me at least share with you the clue I received from Markhti Tarkhil, age 104, of Duripshi in Abkhasia. Markhti told me that every morning as long as he can remember he walks half a mile down a steep hill to bathe in the icy waters of a rapid mountain stream. After dressing he climbs back up the hill to his house. Surely any day Markhti can do that he must be too fit to die. The next day he repeats this physical activity, and so on, day after day while the years roll by—and at 104 Markhti is still much too fit to die!

BIBLIOGRAPHY

GENERAL

Birren, J. E., ed.: *Handbook of Aging and the Individual: Psychological and Biological Aspects.* University of Chicago Press, 1959.

Busse, E. W., and Jeffers, F. C., eds.: Proceedings of Seminars 1965–69: Duke University Council on Aging and Human Development. Duke University Medical Center, Durham, North Carolina, 1969.

Busse, E. W., and Pfeiffer, E., eds.: *Behavior and Adaption in Late Life.* Little, Brown and Company, Boston, 1969.

Comfort, A.: *Ageing: The Biology of Senescence.* Holt, Rinehart and Winston, Inc., New York, 1964.

Comfort, A.: Test-battery to measure ageing-rate in man. *Lancet, 2:* 1411–1415, 1969.

Goldstein, S.: The biology of aging. *N. Eng. J. Med., 285:* 1120–1129, 1971.

Krohn, P. L. ed.: *Topics in the Biology of Aging.* Interscience, New York, 1966.

Rosenfeld, A.: The longevity seekers. *Saturday Review of the Sciences,* 47–51, March 1973.

Shock, N. W., ed.: *Perspectives in Experimental Gerontology.* Charles C. Thomas, Publisher, Springfield, Illinois, 1966.

Strehler, B. L., ed: *Time, Cells and Aging.* Academic Press, New York, 1962.

Strehler, B. L., ed.: *Advances in Gerontological Research.* Academic Press, New York, Vol. 1, 1964; Vol. 2, 1967; Vol. 3, 1971; Vol. 4, 1972.

Verzar, F.: *Experimentelle Gérontologie.* Ferdinand Enke Verlag, Stuttgart, 1965.

Woolhouse, H. W., ed.: *Aspects of the Biology of Ageing.* Cambridge University Press, New York, 1967.

Woolhouse, H. W., ed.: *Symposia of the Society for Experimental Biology—Aspects of the Biology of Ageing. 21.* Academic Press, Inc., New York, 1967.

INTRODUCTIONS

Leaf, A.: Everyday is a gift when you are over 100. *National Geographic, 143:* 93–119, 1973.

Leaf, A.: Getting old. *Sci. Amer., 229*: 45–52, 1973.

Leaf, A.: Unusual longevity: the common denominators. *Hosp. Prac., 8:* 75–86, 1973.

Silverberg, E., and Holleb, A. I.: Cancer statistics. *Ca-A Cancer J. for Clinicians, 23:* 2–27, 1973.

Simon, A. B., and Alonzo, A. A.: Sudden death in nonhospitalized cardiac patients. *Arch. Int. Med., 132*: 163–170, 1973.

I THE CAUCASUS

Benet, S.: *Abkhasia: The Long-Living People of the Caucasus.* Holt, Rinehart and Winston, Inc., New York, 1974.

Chebotarev, D. F., and Sachuk, Nina N.: Sociomedical examination of longevous people in the USSR. *J. Geront., 19:* 435–439, 1964.

Guinness Book of World Records, 1974. Sterling Publishing Company, New York, pp. 25–29.

McKain, Walter C.: Are they really that old? *Gerontologist, 7:* 70–80, 1967.

Myers, R. J.: Economic security in the Soviet Union. *Trans. Soc. Actuaries, 11:* 723–724, 745, 1959.

Myers, R. J.: Further analysis of Soviet data on mortality and fertility. *Public Health Reports, 77:* 177–182, 1962.

Myers, R. J.: Comparative analysis of mortality in the Soviet Union. *International Population Conference,* New York, 2 vols., 35–42, 1963.

Myers, R. J.: Analysis of mortality in the Soviet Union according to 1958–59 life tables. *Trans. Soc. Actuaries; 16:* 309–317, 1964.

II HUNZA

Ali, S. M.: A nutritional survey in Hunza. *Pakistan J. Med. Research, 5:* 141–147, April 1966.

Clark, J.: *Hunza: Lost Kingdom of the Himalayas.* Funk & Wagnalls Company, New York, 1956.

Douglas, W. O.: Book review: *Lost Kingdom of the Himalayas* by J. Clark, *Saturday Review 39:* 18, June 2, 1956.

Haider, R., and Ahmad, G.: Health and longevity in Hunza. *Pakistan J. Med. Research, 5:* 133–140, April 1966.

Khan, S. A., and Bhatty, M. K.: Fats in Hunza diets in relation to their life span. *Pakistan J. Med. Research, 5:* 169–175, April 1966.

Levine, S. A., and Vathur, V. S.: A brief survey of the health of aged Hunzas. *Annotations, 68:* 841, 1973.

Lorimer, E. O.: *Language Hunting in the Karakoram.* George Allen & Unwin, Ltd., London, 1939.

McCarrison, Sir Robert: *Nutrition and Health.* The Cantor Lectures, Faber & Faber, Ltd., London, 1936.

Shah, F. H., Salam, A., Javaid, J. I., and Hamid, A.: The nutritive value of Hunza foods. *Pakistan J. Med. Research, 5:* 148–159, April 1966.

Shah, F. H., Qureshi, M. A., and Salam, A.: Chemical and microbiological studies of Hunza water and wine. *Pakistan J. Med. Research, 5:* 160–168, April 1966.

III VILCABAMBA

Salvador M. y Colaboradores: *Vilcabamba: Tierra de Longevos. Casa de la Cultura Ecuadoriana, Quito, 1972.*

V NUTRITION

Ahrens, R. A.: Sucrose, hypertension and heart disease: an historical perspective. *Am. J. Clin. Nutrition, 27:* 403–422, 1974.

Are PUFA harmful? Selections from the *Brit. Med. J., 4:* 1–2, 5–6, 1973.

Armstrong, M. L., Warner, E. D., and Connor, W. E.: Regression of coronary atheromatosis in rhesus monkeys. *Circ. Res., 27:* 59–67, 1970.

Benditt, Earl P., and Benditt, John M.: Evidence for a monoclonal origin of human atherosclerotic placques. *Proc. Nat. Acad. Sci., 70:* 1753–1756, 1973.

Bierenbaum, M. L., Fleischman, A. I., Green, D. P., Raichelson, R. I., Hayton, T., Watson, P. B., and Caldwell, A. B.: The 5-year experience of modified fat diets on younger men with coronary heart disease. *Circulation, 52:* 943–952, 1970.

Biss, K., Ho, K-J., Mikkelson, B., Lewis, L., and Taylor, C. B.: Some unique biologic characteristics of the Masai of East Africa. *N. Eng. J. Med, 284:* 694–699, 1971.

Blumenthal, S., and Jesse, M. J.: Prevention of atherosclerosis: a pediatric problem. *Hosp. Prac., 8:* 81–90, 1973.

Burkitt, D. P.: Some diseases characteristic of modern Western civilization. *Brit. Med. J., 1:* 274–278, 1973.

Christakis, G., Rinzler, S. H., Archer, M., Winslow, G., Jampel, S., Stephenson, J., Friedman, G., Fein, H., Kraus, A., and James, G.: The anti-coronary club: a dietary approach to the prevention of coronary heart disease—a seven-year report. *Am. J. Public Health, 56:* 299–314, 1966.

Controlled trial of a soya-bean oil in myocardial infarction. Report of a research committee to the Medical Research Council. *Lancet, 2:* 693–699, 1968.

Dahl, L. K.: Salt and hypertension. *Am. J. Clin. Nutrition, 25:* 231–244, 1972.

Dayton, S., et al: Controlled trial of a diet high in unsaturated fat for prevention of atherosclerotic complications. *Lancet, 2:* 1060–1062, 1968.

Dietschy, J. M., and Wilson, J. D.: Regulation of cholesterol metabolism. *N. Eng. J. Med., 282:* 1128–2238, 1970.

Ederer, F., Leren, P., Turpeinen, S., and Frantz, I. D., Jr.: Cancer among men on cholesterol-lowering diets. *Lancet, 2:* 203–207, 1971.

Food intake and nutritive value of diets of men, women, and children in the United States, Spring of 1965. *Agricultural Research Service,* 62–18, March 1969.

Fredrickson, D. S., and Levy, R. I.: Familial hyperlipoproteinemia. Chapter 28 in *The Metabolic Basis of Inherited Disease,* ed. by Stanbury, J. B., Wyngaarden, J. B., and Fredrickson, D. S., 545–614, 3rd ed. McGraw-Hill, New York, 1972.

Goldstein, J. L., Schrott, H. G., Hazzard, W. R., Bierman, E. L., and Motulsky, A. G.: Hyperlipidemia in coronary heart disease. II. Genetic analysis of lipid levels in 1976 families and delineation of a new inherited disorder, combined hyperlipidemia. *J. Clin. Invest., 52:* 1544–1568, 1973.

Goldstein, J. L., Schrott, H. G., Hazzard, W. R., Bierman, E. L., and Motulsky, A. G.: Hyperlipidemia in coronary heart disease. III. Evaluation of lipoprotein phenotypes of 156 genetically defined survivors of myocardial infarction. *J. Clin. Invest., 52:* 1569–1577, 1973.

Gordon, T., and Kannel, W. B.: Predisposition to atherosclerosis in the head, heart, and legs. *J. A. M. A., 221:* 661–666, 1972.

Gordon, T., and Kannel, W. B.: The effects of overweight on cardiovascular diseases. *Geriatrics, 28:* 80–88, 1973.

Heaton, K. W.: Food fibre as an obstacle to energy intake. *Lancet, 2:* 1418–1421, 1973.

Hirsch, J., and Knittle, J. L.: Cellularity of obese and non-obese human adipose tissue. *Fed. Proc., 29:* 1516–1521, 1970.

Hirsch, J.: Can we modify the number of adipose cells? *Postgrad. Med., 51:* 83–86, 1972.

Johnson, P. R., Zucker, L. M., Cruce, J. A. F., and Hirsch, J.: Cellularity of adipose depots in the genetically obese Zucker rat. *J. Lipid Res., 12:* 706–714, 1971.

Johnson, P. R. and Hirsch, J.: Cellularity of adipose depots in six strains of genetically obese mice. *J. Lipid Res., 13:* 2–11, 1972.

Jose, D. G., and Good, R. A.: Quantitative effects of nutritional essential amino acid deficiency upon immune responses to tumors in mice. *J. Exp. Med., 137:* 1–9, 1973.

Jose, D. G.: The cancer connection with immunity and nutrition. *Nutrition Today,* pp. 4–9, March–April 1973.

Kannel, W. B., Dawber, T. R., Friedman, G. D., Glennon, W. E., and McNamara, P. M.: Risk factors in coronary heart disease: an evaluation of several serum lipids as predictors of coronary heart disease. *Ann. Int. Med., 61:* 888–899, 1964.

Keys, A., et al: Probability of middle-aged men developing coronary heart disease in five years. *Circulation, 65:* 815–827, 1972.

Leren, P.: The effect of plasma cholesterol lowering diet in male survivors of myocardial infarction. A controlled clinical trial. *Acta Med. Scand.,* Supp. 466, pp. 1–92, 1966.

Leren, P.: The Oslo diet-heart study. Eleven-year report. *Circulation, 42:* 935–942, 1970.

Lewis, B., Wootton, I. D. P., Krikler, D. M., February, A., Chait, A., Oakley, C. M., Sigurdsson, G., Maurer, B., and Birkhead, J.: Frequency of risk factors for ischaemic heart disease in a healthy British population. *Lancet, 2:* 141–146, 1974.

Mann, G. V.: The influence of obesity on health. *N. Eng. J. Med., 291:* 178–185, 226–232, 1974.

Mayer, J.: *Health.* W. B. Saunders Company, Philadelphia, 1974.

McCay, C. M., Maynard, L. A., Sperling, G., and Barnes, L. L.: Retarded growth, life span, ultimate body size and age changes in the albino rat after feeding diets restricted in calories. *J. Nutr., 18:* 1, 1939.

McCay, C. M.: in: Lansing, A. I., ed., *Problems of Ageing.* The Williams & Wilkins Company, Baltimore, 1952.

Miettinen, M., Karvonen, M. J., Turpeinen, O., Elosuo, R., and Paavilainen, E.: Effect of cholesterol-lowering diet on mortality from coronary heart disease and other causes. *Lancet 2:* 835–838, 1972.

Pearce, M. L., and Dayton, S.: Incidence of cancer in men on a diet high in polyunsaturated fat. *Lancet 1:* 464–467, 1971.

Schlenker, E. D., Feurig, J. S., Stone, L. H., Ohlson, M. A., and Mickelsen, O.: Nutrition and health of older people. *Am. J. Clin. Nutr. 26:* 1111–1119, 1973.

Turpeinen, O., et al: Dietary prevention of coronary heart disease: long-term experiment. *Am. J. Clin. Nutr., 21:* 255–276, 1968.

Turpeinen, O.: Diet and coronary events. *J. Am. Dietetic Assoc., 52*: 209–213, 1968.

Wilson, W. S., Hulley, S. B., Burrows, M. I., and Nichaman, M. Z.: Serial lipid and lipoprotein responses to the American Heart Association fat-controlled diet. *Am. J. Med., 51:* 491–503, 1971.

Wissler, R. W.: Development of the atherosclerotic plaque, *Hosp. Pract., 8:* 61–72, 1973.

VI PHYSICAL ACTIVITY

Cassel, J. C.: Evans County cardiovascular and cerebrovascular epidemiologic study. *Arch. Int. Med., 128:* 883–986, 1971.

Epstein, S. E., Redwood, D. R., Goldstein, R. E., Beiser, G. D., Rosing, D. R., Glancy, D. L., Reis, R. L., and Stinson, E. B.: Angina pectoris: pathophysiology, evaluation and treatment. *Ann. Int. Med., 75:* 263–296, 1971.

Morris, J. N., Heady, J. A., Raffle, P. A. B., Roberts, C. G., and Parks, J. W.: Coronary heart disease and physical activity of work. *Lancet, 2:* 1053–1057, 1953.

Morris, J. N., Heady, J., Raffle P. A. B., Roberts, C. G., and Parks, J. W.: Coronary heart disease and physical activity of work. II. Statement and testing of provisional hypothesis. *Lancet 2:* 1111–1120, 1953.

Morris, J. N., and Crawford, M. D.: Coronary heart disease and physical activity of work. Evidence of a national necropsy survey. *Brit. Med. J., 2:* 1485–1496, 1958.

Morris, J. N., Adam, C., Chave, S. P. W., Sirey, C., and Epstein, L.: Vigorous exercise in leisure time and the incidence of coronary heart disease. *Lancet, 1:* 333–339, 1973.

Rose, G., Prineas, J. R., and Mitchell, J. R. A.: Myocardial infarction and the intrinsic calibre of coronary arteries. *Brit. Heart J., 29:* 548–552, 1967.

Stoedefalke, K. G.: Physical fitness programs for adults. *Am. J. Cardiology, 33:* 787–790, 1974.

VII GENETICS

Abbott, M. H., Murphy, E. A., Bolling, D. R., and Abbey, H.: The familial component in longevity. A study of offspring of nonagenarians. II. Preliminary analysis of the completed study. *Johns Hopkins Med. J., 134:* 1–16, 1974.

Dublin, L. I., and Marks, H. H.: The inheritance of longevity—a study based upon life insurance records. 52nd Annual Meeting of the Association of Life Insurance Medical Directors of America, Oct. 23–24, 1941.

Fredrickson, D. S., and Levy, R. I.: Familial hyperlipoproteinemia. Chapter 28 in *The Metabolic Basis of Inherited Disease,* ed. by

Stanbury, J. B., Wyngaarden, J. B., and Fredrickson, D. S., pp. 545–614, 3rd ed., McGraw-Hill, New York, 1972.

Jarvik, L. F.: Genetic aspects of aging. Chapter 4 in *Clinical Geriatrics,* ed. by Isadore Rossman, J. B. Lippincott Company, Philadelphia, pp. 85–105, 1971.

Kallman, F. J., and Jarvik, L. F.: in *Handbook of Aging and the Individual,* ed. by Birren. J. E., University of Chicago Press, 1959.

Larsson, T., Sjogren, T., and Jacobson, G.: Senile dementia. A clinical, sociomedical and genetic study. *Acta Psychiat. Scand., 39:* 1, Suppl. 167, 1963.

Madigan, F. C., and Vance, R. B.: Differential sex mortality: a research design. *Social Forces, 35:* 193, 1957.

VIII SEX AND AGE

Kinsey, A. C., Pomeroy, W. B., and Martin, C. E.: *Sexual Behavior in the Human Male.* W. B. Saunders Company, Philadelphia, 804 pp., 1948.

Kinsey, A. C., Pomeroy, W. B., Martin, C. E., and Gebhard, P. H.: *Sexual Behavior in the Human Female.* W. B. Saunders Company, Philadelphia, 841 pp., 1953.

Masters, W. H., and Johnson, V. E.: *Human Sexual Response.* Little, Brown and Company, Boston, 1966.

Pfeiffer, E.: Sexual behavior in old age. Chapter 8 in *Behavior and Adaptation in Late Life,* ed. by Busse, E. W., and Pfeiffer, E., Little, Brown and Company, Boston, 1969.

IX THE BRAIN AND AGING

Reitan, R. M.: Measurement of psychological changes in aging. In *Duke University Council on Aging and Human Development. Proceedings of Seminars 1965–1969,* ed. by Busse, E. W., and Jeffers, F. C. Center for the Study of Aging and Human Development. Duke University Medical Center, Durham, North Carolina, November 1969.

Reed, H. B. C., and Reitan, R. M.: A comparison of the effects of the normal aging process with the effects of organic brain damage on adaptive abilities. *J. Geront., 18:* 177–179, 1963.

Wisniewski, H. M., and Terry, R. D.: Morphology of the aging brain, human and animal. *Prog. in Brain Res., 40:* 167–186, 1973.

Wisniewski, H. M., and Terry, R. D.: Reexamination of the pathogenesis of the senile plaque. *Prog. in Neuropathology, 2:* 1–26, 1973.

X PSYCHOLOGICAL AND SOCIAL FACTORS

Busse, E. W., and Pfeiffer, E.: Functional psychiatric disorders in old age. In: *Behavior and Adaptation in Late Life,* ed. by Busse, E. W., and Pfeiffer, E. Little, Brown and Company, Boston, pp. 183–235, 1969.

Friedman, M., and Rosenman, R. H.: *Type A Behavior and Your Heart.* Alfred A. Knopf, Inc., 276 pp., 1974.

Jenkins, C. D., Zyzanski, S. J., and Rosenman, R. H.: Progress toward validation of a computer-scored test for the type A coronary-prone behavior pattern. *Psychosomatic Med., 33:* 193–202, 1971.

King, H.: Health in the medical and other learned professions. *J. Chron. Dis., 22:* 257–281, 1969.

Lehr, I., Messinger, H. B., and Rosenman, R. H.: A sociobiological approach to the study of coronary heart disease. *J. Chron. Dis., 26:* 13–30, 1972.

Poskanzer, D. C., Munford, R. S., Williams, S. V., Colton, T., and Murphy, D.: Mortality among physicians: a cohort study. *J. Chron. Dis., 24:* 18–23, 1971.

XI RESEARCH ON AGING

Anderson, R. E.: Longevity in radiated human populations, with particular reference to the atomic bomb survivors. *Am. J. Med., 55:* 643–656, 1973.

Belsky, J. L., Tachikawa, K., and Jablon, S.: The health of atomic bomb survivors: a decade of examinations in a fixed population. *Yale J. Biol. and Med., 46:* 284–296, 1973.

Bjorksten, J.: The crosslinkage theory of aging. *J. Am. Geront. Soc., 16:* 408–427, 1968.

Burnet, F. M.: A genetic interpretation of ageing. *Lancet, 2:* 480–484, 1973.

Cleaver, J. E.: Xeroderma Pigmentosum: a human disease in which an initial stage of DNA repair is defective. *Proc. Nat. Acad. Sci. U.S.A., 63:* 428–435, 1969.

Curtis, H. J.: Biological mechanisms underlying the aging process. *Science, 141:* 686–694, 1963.

Danes, B. S.: Progeria: a cell culture study on aging. *J. Clin. Invest., 50:* 2000–2003, 1971.

Daniel, C. W., Young, L. J. T., Medina, D., and DeOme, K. B.: The influence of mammogenic hormones on serially transplanted mouse mammary gland. *Exp. Geront., 6:* 95–101, 1971.

Dell'orco, R. T., Mertens, J. G., and Kruse, P. F., Jr.: Doubling potential, calendar time, and senescence of human diploid cells in culture. *Exp. Cell Res., 77:* 356–360, 1973.

Epstein, J., Williams, J. R., and Little, J. B.: Deficient DNA repair in human progeroid cells. *Proc. Nat. Acad. Sci. U.S.A., 70:* 977–981, 1973.

Goldstein, S., Littlefield, J. W., and Soeldner, J. S.: Diabetes mellitus and aging: diminished plating efficiency of cultured human fibroblasts. *Proc. Nat. Acad. Sci. U.S.A., 64:* 155–160, 1969.

Goldstein, S.: The role of DNA repair in aging of cultured fibroblasts from Xeroderma Pigmentosum and normals. *Proc. Soc. Exp. Biol. Med., 137:* 730–734, 1971.

Goldstein, S.: The biology of aging. *N. Eng. J. Med., 285:* 1120–1129, 1971.

Greenberg, L. J., and Yunis, E. J.: Immunologic control of aging: a possible primary event. *Gerontologia, 18:* 247–266, 1972.

Hamlin, C. R., and Kohn, R. R.: Determination of human chronological age by study of a collagen sample. *Exp. Geront., 7:* 377–379, 1972.

Harman, D.: Free radical theory of aging: effect of free radical reaction inhibitors in the mortality rate of male LAF mice. *J. Geront., 23:* 476–482, 1968.

Harman, D.: Free radical theory of aging: effect of the amount and degree of unsaturation of dietary fat on mortality rate. *J. Geront., 26:* 451–457, 1971.

Hayflick, L., and Moorhead, P. S.: The serial cultivation of human diploid cell strains. *Exp. Cell Res., 25:* 585–621, 1961.

Hayflick, L.: The limited in vitro lifetime of human diploid cell strains. *Exp. Cell Res., 37:* 611–636, 1965.

Hayflick, L.: Human cells and aging. *Sci. Amer., 218:* 32–37, 1968.

Hayflick, L.: Aging under glass. *Exp. Geront., 5:* 291–303, 1970.

Hayflick, L.: The biology of human aging. *Am. J. Med. Sci., 265:* 432–445, 1973.

Hayflick, L.: The strategy of senescence. *Gerontologist, 14:* 37–45, 1974.

Hayflick, L.: The longevity of cultured human cells. *J. Am. Geriatrics Soc., 22:* 1–12, 1974.

Heidrick, M. L., and Makinodan, T.: Nature of cellular deficiencies in age-related decline of the immune system. *Gerontologia, 18:* 305–320, 1972.

Holliday, R., and Tarrant, G. M.: Altered enzymes in ageing human fibroblasts. *Nature, 238:* 26–30, 1972.

Jose, D. G., and Good, R. A.: Quantitative effects of nutritional essential amino acid deficiency upon immune responses to tumors in mice. *J. Exp. Med., 137:* 1–9, 1973.

Kohn, H. T., and Guttman, P. H.: Age at exposure and the late effects of X-rays; survival and tumor incidence in CAF mice irradiated at 1 to 2 years of age. *Radiation Res., 18:* 348–373, 1963.

Kohn R. R.: Effect of antioxidants on life-span of C57BL mice. *J. Geront., 26:* 378–380, 1971.

Liu, R. K., and Walford, R. L.: The effect of lowered body temperature on lifespan and immune and non-immune processes. *Gerontologia, 18:* 363–388, 1972.

Mackay, I. R.: Ageing and immunological function in man. *Gerontologia, 18:* 285–304, 1972.

Martin, G. M., Sprague, C. A. and Epstein, C. J.: Replicative life-span of cultivated human cells. *Lab. Invest., 23:* 86–92, 1970.

Medvedev, Z. A.: Possible role of repeated nucleotide sequences in DNA in the evolution of life spans of differentiated cells. *Nature, 237:* 453–454, 1972.

Merz, G. S., and Ross, J. D.: Viability of human diploid cells as a function of in vitro age. *J. Cell Physiol., 74:* 219–222, 1969.

Orgel, L. E.: The maintenance of the accuracy of protein synthesis and its relevance to ageing. *Proc. Nat. Acad. Sci. U.S.A., 49:* 517, 1963.

Orgel, L. E.: Ageing of clones of mammalian cells. *Nature, 243:* 441–445, 1973.

Price, G. B., and Makinodan, T.: Aging: alteration of DNA-protein information. *Gerontologia, 19:* 58–70, 1973.

Setlow, R. B., Regan, J. D., German, J., and Carrier, W. L.: Evidence that Xeroderma Pigmentosum cells do not perform the first step in the repair of ultraviolet damage to their DNA. *Proc. Nat. Acad. Sci. U.S.A., 64:* 1035–1041, 1969.

von Hahn, H. P.: Failures of regulation mechanisms as causes of cellular aging. Chapter 1 in: *Advances in Gerontological Research,* Vol. 3, ed. by Bernard L. Strehler, Academic Press, New York, pp. 1–38, 1971.

Walford, R. L.: *The Immunologic Theory of Aging.* Munksgaard, Copenhagen, 1969.

Waters, H., and Walford, R. L.: Latent period for outgrowth of human skin explants as a function of age. *J. Geront., 25:* 381–383, 1970.

Williamson, A. R., and Askonas, B. A.: Senescence of an antibody-forming cell clone. *Nature, 238:* 337–339, 1972.

XIII DO'S AND DONT'S

Dublin, L. I., and Marks, H. H.: The inheritance of longevity—a study based upon life insurance records. Association of Life Insurance Medical Directors of America, pp. 3–34. Press of Recording and Statistical Corporation, New York, 1942.

Ferris, P.: The fountain of youth, updated, in *New York Times Magazine,* Dec. 2, 1973, p. 38.

Graham, S., and Levin, M. L.: Smoking withdrawal in the reduction of risk of lung cancer. *Cancer, 27:* 865–871, 1971.

Lew, E. A.: High blood pressure, other risk factors and longevity: the insurance viewpoint. *Am. J. Med., 55:* 281–194, 1973.

Pearl, R., and Pearl, R. de W.: *The Ancestry of the Long-lived.* Humphrey Milford, London, 1934.

"Risko." In *Lancet, 2:* 243–244, 1973.

Silverberg, E., and Holleb, A. I.: Cancer statistics. *Ca-A Cancer J. for Clinicians, 23:* 1–27, 1973.

Turner, R.: Prevention of coronary heart disease. *Lancet, 2:* 1137–1140, 1973.

U.S. Department of Commerce: Current Population Reports—Special Studies. Some demographic aspects of aging in the U.S., No. 43, pp. 1–30, February 1973.

Woodhall, B., and Jablon, S.: Prospects for further increase in average longevity. *Geriatrics, 12:* 586, 1957.

INDEX

INDEX